HORMONE REPLACEMENT THERAPY
YES OR NO?

HOW TO MAKE AN INFORMED DECISION

about
ESTROGEN, PROGESTERONE,
& OTHER STRATEGIES FOR
DEALING WITH PMS,
MENOPAUSE, & OSTEOPOROSIS

*A new solution to the estrogen
replacement therapy dilemma*

by Betty Kamen, Ph.D.

N_E

Nutrition Encounter, Inc., Novato, California

All of the facts in this book have been very carefully researched and have been drawn from the scientific literature. In no way, however, are any of the suggestions meant to take the place of advice given by physicians. Please consult a medical or health professional should the need for one be indicated.

Nutrition Encounter, Inc., 1993
Box 5847
Novato, CA 94948

Printed in the United States of America
First Printing: 1993
Second Printing: 1993
ISBN 0-944501-07-9

Dedicated to

John R. Lee, M.D.

whose rare vision
has made optimal health
a reality
for many women,
regardless of age

CONTENTS

Figures

Tables

OTHER BOOKS BY BETTY KAMEN, PH.D.

Total Nutrition During Pregnancy:
How To Be Sure You and Your Baby
Are Eating the Right Stuff

Total Nutrition for Breast-Feeding Mothers

Kids Are What They Eat:
What Every Parent Needs to Know About Nutrition

In Pursuit of Youth: Everyday Nutrition

Osteoporosis:
What It Is, How to Prevent It, How to Stop It

Nutrition In Nursing: The New Approach
A Handbook of Nursing Science

Sesame: The Superfood Seed
How It Can Add Vitality To Your Life

Siberian Ginseng:
Up-To-Date Research on the Fabled Tonic Herb

Germanium: A New Approach to Immunity

Startling New Facts About Osteoporosis:
Why Calcium Alone Does Not Prevent Bone Disease

The Chromium Diet, Supplement & Exercise Strategy

New Facts About Fiber:
How Fiber Supplements Can Enhance Your Health

Everything You Always Wanted to Know About Potassium
But Were Too Tired to Ask

Betty Kamen is an award-winning photojournalist with graduate degrees in psychology and nutrition education. She is an internationally-known lecturer, radio/TV host, and author of many major books, hundreds of articles, and several tapes on various aspects of health and nutrition. For many years she hosted *Nutrition 57* on WMCA in New York; *Nutrition Dialogue,* SPN Cable Network; followed by *Nutrition Watch* on KNBR in San Francisco.

ACKNOWLEDGMENTS

Research & chart development
    Paul Kamen

Support and commitment
    Si Kamen
    Perle Kinney

Medical expertise
    Serafina Corsello, M.D.
    Martin Milner, N.D.
    Michael Rosenbaum, M.D.
    Richard Kunin, M.D.
    Robert Atkins, M.D.
    Jerilynn Prior, M.D.
    Katherina Dalton, M.D.

Feedback
    Bernice Goldmark, Ph.D.
    Diana Hanssen

Editing
    Penny Post
    Theresa James Kamen

Cover Design
    Raylene Buehler

Graphic Arts
    New Vision Technologies, Inc.
    TechPool Studios
    ProArt Multi Ad Services
    T/Maker Company
    Wheeler Arts

FOREWORD

Hormone Replacement Therapy: Yes or No? is a profoundly valuable educational resource for women in the twenty-first century. At last, there is a reference that clearly and effectively educates women about their own hormones and body chemistry. Women have finally been given the information, tools, and resources they need to make informed decisions about their own endocrine balance.

As a result of this work, women can be self-empowered to take control of their decisions and treatment options concerning hormone replacement and lifestyle adjustment.

In the ten years of my practice of treating women with natural progesterone and lifestyle changes for the management of PMS and menopause, I have searched far and wide for a definitive reference for patients—one that is thorough, up to date, and in language that the general public can understand. Dr. Kamen's book is the arrival of that resource.

A multiplicity of commonly-held fallacies are replaced with facts, offering the reader a range of options. These include the use of natural progesterone as an alternative to synthetic progestins and the integration of progesterone therapy into an existing estrogen therapy program.

Betty has done a wonderful job of presenting relatively complex endocrine biochemistry in terminology that anyone can understand.

The book invites the general public to sit down and enjoy a reading interlude that cannot help but foster a deep conviction in one's inherent self-healing abilities with the aid of nutrition, lifestyle adjustment, and natural hormone replacement therapies.

So hold on to your seats and get ready for an eye-opening experience into the truth surrounding hormone replacement therapy!

Martin Milner, N.D.
Medical Director, Center for Natural Medicine,
Portland, Oregon
Associate Professor of Cardiovascular and Pulmonary
Medicine at National College of Naturopathic Medicine

AUTHOR'S NOTES

Hippocrates associated the consumption of high-fiber foods with better elimination. But the world didn't pay much attention until Dr. Denis Burkitt made the same "revolutionary" statement in 1980.

Why did it take more than two thousand years from observation to acceptance to practice? Part of the reason can be related to the natural lag that exists between research and application. Part of the reason is the "be-not-the-first-to-try-the-new" paradigm—causing a built-in delay. And part of the reason may be inexplicable human behavior.

Impressed with the benefits of yogurt, Dr. Smith taught several of his patients how to make it. Two days later, one patient called and said, "Dr. Smith, my yogurt turned green!" Dr. Smith answered, "You must have done something wrong." When a second patient called with the same problem, Dr. Smith responded, "Well, that can happen sometimes." After the third call with a similar complaint, Smith retorted, "Oh, yes, that's to be expected."

And so it is with other scientific observations. The medical community is rather skeptical at first, but as results are repeated, everyone finally agrees and says, "We knew that all along." Sometimes it takes twenty centuries, but the average lag is from 40 to 75 years in today's time.

Long before the advent of double-blind, controlled research, doctors learned from clinical experience. The intuitive, astute physician still does!

It is gratifying to me to reflect on ideas that I have presented along the way, and then to find that my conclusions and those of other researchers like myself are validated years later. I anticipate that the core of information presented in this book will have a similar history.

Hopefully, we will not have to wait too long for more physicians to understand the research on estrogen and hormone replacement therapy. Too many women have sacrificed their sense of control when it comes to making decisions about such therapy. That's okay, provided we don't sacrifice our health as well.

Medicine reflects our culture. High technology should help us to understand our bodies, not be a force for attaining metabolism that is artificial and unnatural.

When the use of natural progesterone becomes common practice, those physicians who have looked at the research and have put this successful therapy in place will be ahead of their time. Lucky are their patients.

Betty Kamen

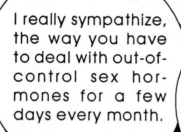
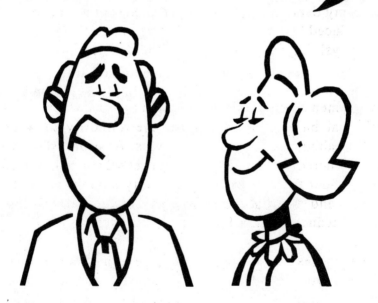

INTRODUCTION

by Serafina Corsello, M.D.

As I was pondering the necessity of writing a book about the hormonal problems of women—from the cradle to the golden years—my dear friend, Betty Kamen, seized the keyboard and produced this most comprehensive, magnificent review of the physiology and pathology of the female reproductive cycle.

Betty Kamen is one of the most prolific medical writers. Her nutritional background gives her the authority to write cogently about the subjects she covers. As usual, she provides an incredible number of references which can be used by the reader for further research. Betty's books are well-indexed and well-documented. She arrives at brilliant medical deductions that I find very enlightening.

Betty proposes the theory that until the turn of the century, very few women suffered the dreadful consequences of hormonal derangement, primarily because of their judicious diet. This is certainly true.

Betty suggests (as I do) that there has been a well-known biased attitude in regard to women's problems. As a physician and a woman, I have had to recognize the subtle discriminatory attitudes that have been so pervasive in the medical field. Until very recently, the male-dominated medical establishment felt much more comfortable relegating women's hormonal problems to the insane asylum, rather than to the benches of biomedical research.

I believe that the heightened interest in research into female reproductive functions will continue because of the economic issues relating to it. In the next twenty years approximately forty million women will enter menopause. No medical establishment, and certainly no pharmaceutical industry, will ignore such a large population and the potential for so much economic return.

Thanks to the leadership of Dr. Bernadine Healy, a most enlightened woman and former Director of the National Institutes of Health, we now have an Institute for Women's Studies, in which women's cardiovascular diseases and hormonal dysfunctions have gained the same importance that male disorders have always received.

Most research, however, focuses solely on estrogen replacement therapy. Very little has been done regarding safe, non-toxic alternatives—which this book so eloquently describes. Unless menopause becomes once again an *uneventful stage of life*, we will be troubled by a plethora of dreadful medical consequences.

We women will be spending *one-third of our lives* in a postmenopausal state. We need to be able to function without becoming plagued by the consequences of poorly-managed menopause.

As a postmenopausal woman, I have had to deal personally with the reality of estrogen replacement therapy. At age fifty-two, with the abrupt onset of insomnia which would not permit me to function at the high level to which I am accustomed, I turned to the "quick fix"—*hormonal replacement therapy*, which includes estrogen and synthetic progesterone.

At age fifty-four, I awoke one morning with an ominous mass in my breast. I had to immediately discontinue the hormones but was faced with the necessity of finding a substitute for them. There was no book such as this to guide me, so I went to the library and read all I could find on the subject of natural, traditional, and Eastern interventions for hot flashes and insomnia—two of the most common symptoms related to these later years.

My newly found knowledge forged the basis of my interest in *natural* replacement therapy. I have since used these interventions on myself and my patients, with great results. Betty's book provides ample tools to assist women in the important task of recognition of the early signs of menopause and what to do about them. (And so much of this information pertains to PMS as well.)

What is menopause? Strictly speaking, it is the time in a woman's life when her menstrual cycle becomes erratic and then stops and estrogen levels fall drastically. There is, however, a transitional stage that can last from five to ten years called *perimenopause.* This phase of our hormonal life is marked by irregularity and "ups and downs" of the hormones along with "ups and downs" of insidious symptoms such as irritability, mood swings, sleep disturbances, changes in memory retention, aches and pains, etc.

The hormonal roller coaster can begin as early as age thirty-five or forty, especially in women who have suffered from PMS, ovarian cysts, endometriosis, and other manifestations of female hormone imbalances.

When the estrogen level abruptly drops—such as in the case of surgical menopause—hot flashes, depression, insomnia, and irritability can be very severe. Statistics tell us that 15 percent of women have absolutely no problem with menopause, 15 percent have severe manifestations, and the rest fall somewhere in between.

Among other things, estrogen regulates the neurotransmitters of the brain—substances which control the function of our nervous system. In this context, estrogen works somewhat like an antidepressant. Thinking processes and motor activity are, in turn, managed by these brain neurotransmitters, which allow brain cells to communicate with each other. Some of the neurotransmitters in question are serotonin, acetylcholine, and gamma butyric acid (commonly referred to as GABA). Proper levels of estrogen help to regulate their uptake or proper function. At the time when estrogen drops, *all hell breaks loose* in predisposed individuals. It is important, therefore, that we women take our destiny in our hands and begin to recognize the early signs of this hormonal imbalance.

One of the first markers is, in fact, irritability. Women often report being besieged by a loosely-defined sense of malaise. They say, "I'm just not the same." In some cases, they fall into a state of bewilderment and depression. These are the women who populate the welcoming couches of psychoanalysts in search of elusive answers.

Another change occurs in the quality and/or quantity of the menstrual flow. All of a sudden a cycle will skip, and the next one may be frighteningly heavy with clots and pain.

With laboratory technology, we can now test certain hormones to establish whether or not we have entered menopause. In the perimenopausal phase, these hormones can be absolutely normal—while subtle but significant imbalances in the overall hormonal patterns are taking place. The perimenopausal phase, for however long it lasts, always ends in menopause, accompanied by total cessation of the menstrual flow. It may also be accompanied by vaginal atrophy, acceleration of the aging process, propensity to cardiovascular disorders, and osteoporosis.

Until there is ovarian failure, the diagnosis is in the art of empathic listening.

I have had to recognize that as sympathetic as I thought I always was, I became a more sensitive, receptive antenna to my patients' subtle perimenopausal problems when I myself went through the experience. Life is the best teacher, but, as our experiences with homogeneous support groups have taught us, this does *not* mean that only people who experience problems can treat them. It only means that they may be able to do it better.

At a time when the body is going through fluctuations of estrogen and progesterone, the sense of instability is understandably worse. This comprehensive book gives wonderful suggestions that can help avoid the unpleasantness associated with the perimenopausal phase of life. Once the storm is over, the *postmenopausal zest*—to quote Margaret Mead—gives us freedom, liberation, and the capacity to function.

Unencumbered by the responsibilities of young women, fear of pregnancy, and care of our children, we can now set out to become what we really are. Postmenopausal liberation can lead to a splendid valley of achievements. My dear friend Betty is a perfect example of this model.

I want to reiterate this point: the worst time is during the perimenopausal-menopausal transitional stage. Once that is over, with the help of suggestions such as the ones contained in this book, the rewards are sizeable. If one can reach the menopausal zest, it can be one of the most rewarding stages of life. As Betty suggests, one "cashes in at the end what one has saved at the beginning."

Unfortunately for us, the beginning may go as far back as our prenatal phase. One of my greatest joys is, in fact, the treatment of infertile women, who, through natural methodology, then become fertile. These women continue to eat well, take adequate nutrients, have a joyous attitude, and deliver what I call "super babies." These babies, if they continue to take good care of themselves throughout their lives, will have none of the problems associated with menopausal "storms."

I have seen patients in whom menopausal symptoms become worse when they take synthetic progestins, as prescribed during hormone replacement therapy. This has convinced me, more than anything else, to put myself and my patients on the kind of program that Betty outlines.

As we enter the age of self-determination, it is up to us to improve our heritage. Women who diet excessively without compensating with proper amounts of vitamins, minerals, and antioxidants are inviting trouble. Decline in bone mass begins very early in life. By age thirty-five, it is already an established fact. Judicious exercise, accompanied by appropriate intake of nutrients and a proper diet (as described in this book), is absolutely the best strategy.

Women with severe PMS can count on difficulties at the end of the road. Treating PMS naturally prevents the difficultly later in life. Menopause then becomes just "the silent passage," as described by Gail Sheehy.

By writing such a cogent and comprehensive book on the natural management of all female hormonal problems, Betty Kamen has given a new lease on life to thousands of women. As a clinician, I can attest to the fact that diet, attitude, and natural interventions do make an *enormous* difference. Betty has written a book that teaches us how to balance all elements of life. She has succeeded in giving a compendium of events that can lead to a safe hormonal voyage. Betty takes us step by step through that journey, illustrating how everything works. The goal is to achieve an easy transition. The result is the attainment of postmenopausal zest.

Congratulations, Betty, and congratulations to your readers.

Serafina Corsello, M.D.
Director, Corsello Centers
New York, New York; Huntington, New York
Member, National Institute of Health,
Office of Alternative Medicine

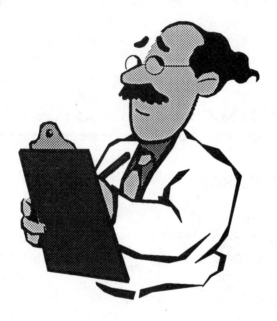

"You want to know if you should go on hormone replacement therapy? Well, yes and no. But don't quote me!"

1

FEMININE AND AFFLICTED

HOW IT IS, HOW IT WAS, HOW IT COULD BE

When I began my research for this book, I was astounded to learn that the first scientific description of what we now call PMS, or premenstrual syndrome, did not appear until 1931. Prior to that time, difficulties relating to menstruation were referred to as premenstrual tension—and even that designation is a product of relatively modern-day classification. The initials PMS did not became part of the medical (and popular) lexicon until 1953, when Katherina Dalton and Raymond Greene published a paper called "The Premenstrual Syndrome." Finally, PMS was recognized as a syndrome—a collection of loosely-related symptoms—described in the medical literature.

Why did it take so long? Hadn't half the population of the world suffered, more or less, with PMS every month of every year for the entire history of the human species? Are we to believe that very few women got PMS before 1931? Or that the variety of symptoms had never been correlated and listed before 1953? After all, hadn't the symptoms of many other significant disorders been recorded with explicit detail over the centuries?

Certainly there's always been a male bias in academic medical research. But even making allowances for possible neglect, it seems incredible that a problem so universal should have received so little attention. Similarly, the focus on the widespread incidence of breast cancer and difficulties related to menopause is a very recent development. Even osteoporosis was unheard of outside the medical profession just a few years ago, yet now it's a household word.

Had these disorders been ignored? Or did doctors have completely different names or different diagnoses for them? What was going on?

The answer is discouragingly simple. The physicians who cared for our grandmothers and great-grandmothers weren't very concerned about PMS, osteoporosis, menopausal problems, or breast cancer *because our grandmothers and great-grandmothers weren't very concerned about them, either.* Menstrual- and menopause-related problems just didn't come up that often among our naturally-nourished ancestors. Yet in this century we have come to accept these irregularities as part of being female—a universal constant of the gender. I seriously question this assumption. Truly healthy women *do not* suffer from these diseases—ever!

Before you dismiss me as a hopeless nutritional idealist, let me add that the conditions of "well-nourished" and "healthy" are admittedly elusive goals that very few women fully achieve in North America. We are all under continuous assault from pollution, exercise deprivation, stress, and, worst of all, the abysmally-poor quality of what we have come to regard as "normal" food, not to mention the effects of poor lighting, environmental chemicals, and the strained ergonomics of the typical indoor workplace!

Compare our current environment with that of only a few generations ago. The daily routine was full of physical activity. The air was clean. Indoor smoke was rare. Chemical solvents were unheard of. Devices that produce stray electromagnetic fields had yet to be invented.

But the biggest difference was the food. Food was full of nutrients and free of pesticides. It was locally produced and genetically unaltered. Most important, it was fresh, and it wasn't junk—no soda, no ice cream, no donuts, no potato chips, no pop tarts—hardly any sugar and not much salt. There were lots of vegetables eaten in season along with freshly-killed meat or freshly-caught fish when it was available. Food was preserved for winter without benefit of a chemical engineer.

> ## Processed food was the exception, not the rule!

You probably still think I'm a hopeless idealist when it comes to food, diet, and health. "Sure," you must be thinking, "as if I can turn back the clock a hundred years and be magically free of all my health problems."

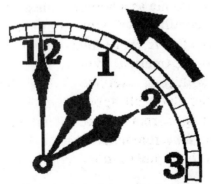

We all know we can't turn the clock back.

Even if we were to swear off the supermarket, the car, and the office forever and walk into the woods to eat nothing but freshly-caught fish, freshly-killed meat (and eat most of it uncooked, while we're at it), and freshly-picked fruits and vegetables, we could never return to the optimal health of people who have lived like that all of their lives. Damage has been done, beginning with our parents' (and possibly our grandparents') lifestyles before we were conceived.

> The effect of nutrition crosses generation lines.

And even if we could turn back that clock, would we really want to give up the convenience of our post-industrial, high-tech lifestyle in pursuit of that last elusive increment of optimal health?

We are left with serious compromises. Although we still have a lot to learn, much is now known about menopause, osteoporosis, PMS, and breast cancer, and there are accepted treatments for all these problems. But there are major differences among the various forms of doctoring and management. Some substances short-circuit our natural healing mechanisms, while others may enhance and promote those very same processes. Most treatments, however, are interventionist—that is, they interfere with our body's natural methods for correcting imbalances.

> Too many of today's medical treatments get in the way of our body's ability to heal itself.

WHAT THIS BOOK IS ABOUT

This book is aimed at examining today's strategies for dealing with PMS, menopause, and osteoporosis and at helping you decide on your personal course of action in these areas. Estrogen replacement therapy in the treatment and prevention of osteoporosis is discussed, as well as natural progesterone as an alternative to that therapy—plus the reasons for the use of certain food supplements. I present my view, which springs from clinical experience, from a broad range of interviews with medical professionals, and from intensive research of published literature.

I want to share with you:

> - facts and fallacies about PMS, menopause, and osteoporosis
> - advantages and disadvantages of estrogen therapy, with emphasis on increasing evidence demonstrating how and why this therapy is harmful
> - advantages and disadvantages of adding synthetic progestins to hormone therapy
> - advantages of adding natural progesterone to hormone therapy
> - the rationale for using natural progesterone *transdermally*
> - the basis for including certain food supplements
> - the justification for specific food cautions

After extensive examination of all sides of the various issues, I have formed fairly strong conclusions. So you will find in these pages that I frequently take positions advocating specific courses of action. Although there is certainly no shortage of controversy, I would be doing you a disservice if I were to avoid passing along my enlightened conclusions, opinions, and even hunches. The sources of the prestigious medical research that I have scrutinized and the details of my interviews with the clinicians—all of which helped bring me to these conclusions—are cited throughout this book.

Simply stated, I am an advocate of using transdermally-applied natural progesterone—along with specific food supplements—as an alternative to more traditional hormone treatments. You should know that I didn't start out with this view. Before my research, I was more inclined to oppose *any* therapy that presumes to improve on nature's own balance of hormones. But without intending to, I assembled a compelling case for natural progesterone. It was difficult to find a single informed source that had anything negative to say about this form of treatment. I'm convinced, and, hopefully, you will be too.

> There is impressive evidence that natural progesterone can correct a critical deficiency which may prove to be the real cause of PMS, menopausal symptoms, and osteoporosis.

Should *you* start using natural progesterone in cream or oil-based form? Should *you* do this instead of taking the estrogen or combined estrogen-progestogen pills that your doctor may be prescribing? Should *you* consume certain supplements on a daily basis? Should *you* proceed without your physician's full cooperation? Should *your physician* read this book? These are the questions answered here.

If it's health you're seeking, or freedom from annoying symptoms, you are not going to get off easy—no matter what your decisions on these issues. The use of natural progesterone, while far safer than alternatives, is still an intervention to be applied only with knowledge and care. And progesterone is only part of the solution, at best. You probably already know that if you want to enjoy *optimal* health, you'll have to give up a few fast-held, fast-food habits. In fact, to be totally unencumbered by annoying discomforts, some of you may have to make what you would consider very substantial sacrifices in your nutritional lifestyle. The point is that such a goal is entirely possible, regardless of your health status.

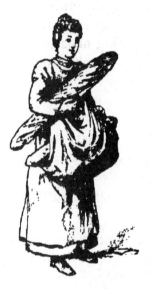

Are we talking about turning back the clock again? No, we can't retreat to the nineteenth century. We don't want to.

But we can pick and choose between knowledge of the past and present and project our future choices based on this wisdom. If we are successful, we'll be able to give PMS, osteoporosis, and menopausal symptoms as little regard as the women and physicians of generations ago.

¤

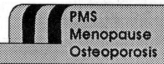

MEMOS

PMS
Menopause
Osteoporosis

➤ Approximately 90 percent of all women in the United States have at least some type of menstrual complaint. For one in ten, symptoms are intensely harsh *and are moderate to severe in up to 40 percent.* Is there any woman who can't relate to the following:

> "Once a month, I feel as though 50 boy scouts are tying knots in my groin."
> "Once a month, a butterfly collection is let loose in my stomach."
> "Once a month, the Music Man's 76 trombones parade around in my head."
> "Yesterday, I spent a year doing routine office work."

➤ Tribal rituals welcoming young girls to womanhood at the start of menstruation were very happy occasions, including song, laughter, and dance. It was considered a sacred time during which women were not to be disturbed. Menstrual taboos were created to protect women.

➤ In more primitive societies today, menstruation is not associated with a syndrome, and fewer women complain of cramps or discomfort than in our advanced culture.[1]

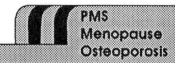

> Several physicians (and many women) confirm that switching to nutrient-dense diets results in the disappearance of PMS.

> Case Western Reserve Medical School discusses the good-health practices of a tribal South African group that is totally free of menopausal symptoms.[2]

> The French *Journal of Obstetrics and Gynecology* reminds us that the nutritional demands for certain nutrients are high during menopause and that the consequences of deficiencies are hormonal disturbances.[3]

> Not all postmenopausal women develop osteoporosis, as pointed out in the German publication, *Wiener Medizinische Wochenschrift*, 1990.[4]

> In 1990, the *Annual Review of Nutrition* noted that when diet, physical activity, cigarette smoking, and alcohol consumption are modified, the usual risks associated with menopause are reduced.[5]

> There are cultures in the world where words for "PMS" or "hot flash" do not exist.

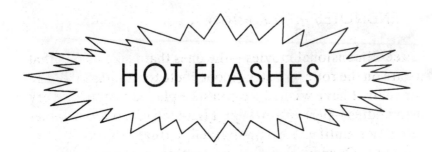

HOT FLASHES

➤ One in three women develops osteoporosis eventually. Low bone mass and structural deterioration leads to fractures.

International Journal of Clinical Pharmacology, Therapy, and Toxicology, 1992[6]

➤ Osteoporosis is expensive and disabling, and the chances of getting it to some degree are almost certain.

Optimal Health Guidelines, 1993[7]

➤ Most "new" diseases are caused by an external agent.

Lancet, 1993[8]

➤ Humans will continue to inflict new diseases on themselves due to environmental changes or even medical intervention.

Lancet, 1993[9]

➤ The recognition of a new disease may be delayed until it is widespread enough and medicine is ready to receive it.

Lancet, 1993[10]

~~ ENDNOTES ~~ *A Fantasy...*

Three-dimensional movies—the ones that make us feel that
we are on the roller coaster—contribute to a fantasy I've had
for years. I have wished we could be placed inside our very
own bodies—perhaps through high-tech simulation, something not unlike a computerized virtual-reality sensory
jumpsuit. Or maybe even with an old-fashioned Aladdin's
lamp. Instead of roller-coaster whirlings through our heads
and stomachs (as in the movies of my youth), we would
encounter a visual sensing of hormonal happenings. *We
would have a direct view of the magic of metabolism.*

I wish we could be witness to the power, the authority, the
wonder of our hormones while their actions are in progress.
Then we would know just how they work and how they
affect our health—for better or for worse.

Since neither our computers nor our science (nor our magic)
have reached that level of sophistication, we must resort to
more conventional modes of learning. The next section
explains some of what we know about hormones—knowledge
that may help us to make our decisions about hormone
replacement therapy.

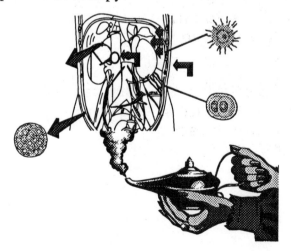

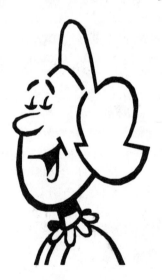

2

WHAT IS A HORMONE?

WHAT HORMONES DO

Hormones control a lot more of your body's functions than just sex. Hormones are secreted by glands—such as your pancreas, adrenal, thyroid, and ovaries—in very small quantities, usually into your blood stream. As they journey around, these powerful substances proceed to activate, control, or direct. No wonder the word hormone is from the Greek *hormaein*, which means *to excite*.

Not consumed as energy (as food is) nor produced as by-products of metabolic processes, hormones are specifically aimed at controlling other processes in your body, often at a location far from where they are produced. Your body does not physically direct a hormone to a particular tissue or organ unless the target is right next to the gland producing the hormone (or is producing the hormone itself). Instead, a hormone travels until it is recognized by a receptor shaped to fit, the way pieces of a jigsaw puzzle fit together.

In Commander-In-Chief style, hormones help some of your cells create protective "coats of armor," guide other cells to trail-blaze, instruct molecular switches to turn on or off, mandate immune processes to grapple with invaders, and charge receptors to stoke fires that require more fuel. They are responsible for glands inducing *differentiation*—prodding a cell which appears to be able to turn into *anything* during the fetal stage, to turn into *something very specific* years, even decades, later.

FIGURE 1

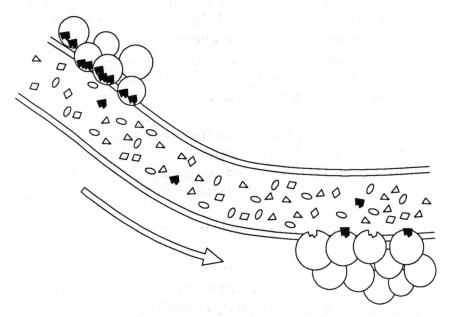

HORMONES: FROM GLAND TO TARGET ORGAN

A small concentration of a hormone can affect tissue at a remote location. The circles at upper left represent cells in a hormone-producing gland. Hormones are represented by the black particles. The hormone enters the bloodstream and will only exit when encountering a matching receptor, as represented by the circles at lower right. Other hormones have no effect on this receptor—they just don't "fit."

Hormones generally spread out evenly throughout your bloodstream, much like a broadcast radio signal. Only certain cells of certain organs or tissues have their chemical receptors "tuned in" to respond to the effects of that particular hormone. (See Figure 1 on page 22.)

It's truly amazing how very few hormone molecules are required to produce a major effect. Even at the top end of the range, there is only one hormone molecule for every *fifty billion* molecules in your blood plasma. At the low end of the concentration sweep, there may be one hundred times fewer hormone molecules—one in every *five zillion* (that's five thousand billion!). *Keep this in mind when you consider intervening by using synthetic hormones in your own body.*

Functionally, hormones can be divided into four categories. There are hormones to control:
    (1) energy production and storage
    (2) water and salt metabolism
    (3) growth
    (4) sexual and reproductive actions

Of course, there's a certain degree of overlap. If it were not for the effects of progesterone and estrogen on the integrity of your bones, for example, you would probably have no reason to be reading this book. The multiple interrelationships between various hormones and other nutrients make the subject interesting but also create controversy for the individual attempting to maintain optimum health. And it can be especially confusing for those whose physicians recommend hormone replacement therapy in *anticipation* of trouble. Many doctors sincerely believe that certain difficulties are inescapable with age. (Fortunately, others do not share this view and have demonstrated its fallacy.)

Your glands manufacture hormones from:
> amino acids
> proteins or peptides
> cholesterol

Hormones made from cholesterol are called *steroid* hormones—the category with which this book is concerned. We often associate the word steroid with the huge muscles adorning men on the covers of sports magazines and the word cholesterol with the "bad" fatty substance found in most animal-derived food (that nasty heart-disease and arteriosclerosis accomplice).

> Steroid hormones play many vital and beneficial roles in human metabolism, just as cholesterol has the important job of serving as a building block for necessary hormones.

Cholesterol's role in heart disease is actually somewhat indirect, and it may not deserve the terrible reputation it has acquired over the last few decades. Interestingly, cholesterol is produced in almost every cell in your body. Your liver spews it out in especially large quantities. The cholesterol in whole foods (in fresh eggs or pure meat, for example) has still not been proved responsible for contributing to the cholesterol build-up that damages arteries. Dietary cholesterol itself may be an innocent bystander, while other factors (such as processed fats in general and even stress) do contribute to excess cholesterol build-up leading to arteriosclerosis.

Figure 2 on page 26 shows a diagram of a cholesterol molecule with some of the other hormone molecules that are made from it. Notice how much of each molecule is identical in each representation. This part of the cholesterol molecule is referred to as the *17-carbon backbone.*

Now notice the relatively subtle modifications of this cholesterol backbone. The minor differences determine which hormone it is.

> The difference between testosterone and one type of estrogen is simply the addition of one hydrogen atom. When one notch on a key is just a little bit different, it opens a completely different lock.

Another factor that distinguishes steroid hormones from other hormones is that they generally cannot be stored inside the cells of the glands that manufacture them. Rather, they are released immediately into your bloodstream as soon as they are produced.

> Since steroid hormones are made from cholesterol, it's important to have an ample supply of cholesterol to work with at all times. Also crucial: an adequate supply of the nutrients producing the enzymes necessary for this hormone synthesis.

FIGURE 2

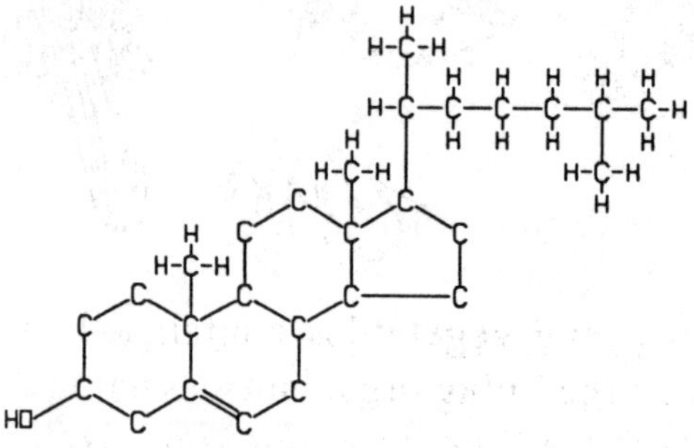

CHOLESTEROL

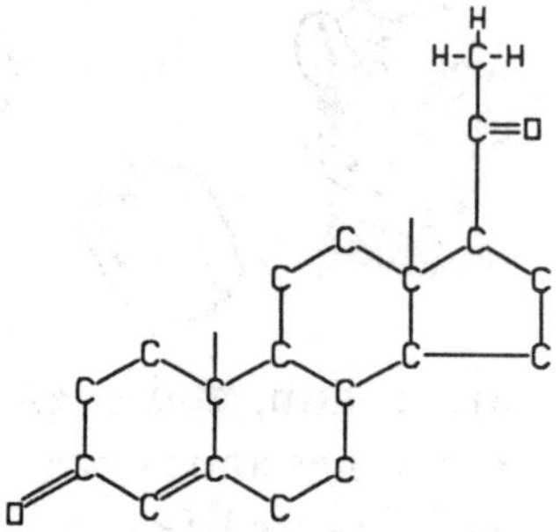

PROGESTERONE

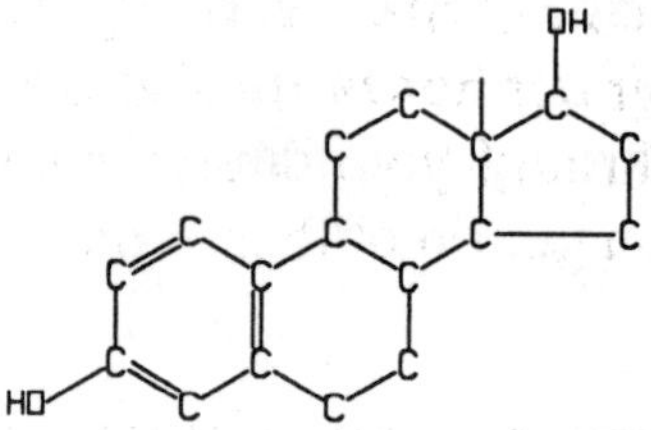

ESTRADIOL
(an estrogen)

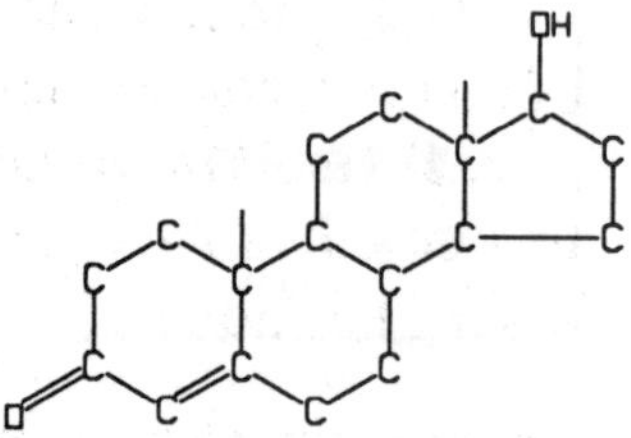

TESTOSTERONE
(an androgen)

THE CHOLESTEROL MOLECULE AND THREE STEROID HORMONES MADE FROM IT

This represents the cholesterol molecule and three steroid hormones that can be manufactured from it by your adrenal cortex. Notice how little difference there is between the androgen *testosterone* and the estrogen *estradiol.*

WHAT HAPPENS WHEN YOU EAT HORMONES?

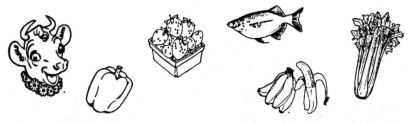

Meat, fish, and even fruits and vegetables contain all the hormones and enzymes that the living organism was using to regulate its life processes at the time it became food. If this blend of chemical signals suddenly becomes mixed with *your* hormones and enzymes, the result would be disastrous—like trying to run a complicated machine with the wrong set of instructions. So immediately after hormones are digested in your small intestines, they pass through your liver, which is pretty smart—your liver helps you get rid of these unnecessary hormones.

> One of your liver's most important functions is to break down the "bad guys," or keep them out of your bloodstream by returning them to your digestive tract.

There's an interesting design feature here: your liver returns the unwanted hormones to your digestive tract at the entrance to your small intestines, where they could get reabsorbed! It's like placing the sewage outlet up-river from where the town gets its drinking water. Did nature miss something at this juncture? No! This method of disposal works because the hormones, *first time around,* are converted by your liver into water-soluble forms. They now bind with other substances, making them difficult to get absorbed through your intestines the *second time around.*

In fact, the materials that render the hormones returning to your digestive tract excretable may also act on newly ingested hormones on their first pass through your intestines. So some ingested hormones don't get absorbed even once.

We have, then, (1) the removal of ingested hormones by your liver, and (2) the chemical environment of your intestines that makes hormone absorption difficult. Given these two factors, only a tiny fraction of dietary female hormones and enzymes normally make it into your bloodstream for general circulation.

Considering your body's sensitivity to very small quantities of hormones, it's easy to understand why first-pass hormone removal is an important function of your liver.

But because of first-pass removal, it is difficult to administer hormones by mouth.

> The big breakthrough in oral contraception was the development of a form of estrogen that could be absorbed readily by your digestive system, making the birth control pill a reality.

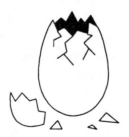

¤

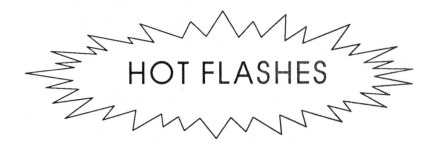

HOT FLASHES

➤ The impact of estrogen on bone metabolism is dependent on how the estrogen is administered.
Journal of Bone and Mineral Research, 1992[1]

➤ Controlled levels of estrogen are difficult *because of first-pass liver metabolism.*
Drugs, 1990[2]

➤ Blood concentrations of estrogen after the same dose vary depending on the mode of administration.[3]
Minerva Endocrinologica, 1989

➤ Undesirable effects of estrogen are hard to avoid when estrogen is taken orally.
Drugs, 1990[4]

➤ Doses of estrogen must be adjusted to achieve desired levels.[5]
Minerva Endocrinologica, 1989

➤ The effectiveness of estrogen is dependent on the dosage and mode of application.
Zentralblatt fur Gynakologie, 1989[6]

➤ After oral application, estrogens always experience the first-pass effect.

Zentralblatt fur Gynakologie, 1989[7]

➤ Fourteen eggs a week do not influence coronary heart-disease risk.

American Journal of Clinical Nutrition, 1992[8]

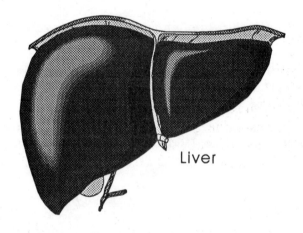

Liver

It has been said that the control panel of a space shuttle is not as complicated as the "control panel" of our liver!

~~ ENDNOTES ~~ *The fantasy continues...*

We watch, wide-eyed, as hormones enter the fast-moving vehicle that transports substances vital to our lives: our bloodstream. We hear the counter clicking away, chalking up the rounds—graphically demonstrating that every single minute, *one thousand four hundred and forty times a day,* our blood circles through our body. We are fascinated by the hormone activity—endless processes taking place concurrently—a three-ring circus, and more.

Some of the work of creating hormones has been farmed out, produced elsewhere—not inside our bodies. These hormones are a little different from those assembled by our own "factories." We observe a synthetic hormone playing the field, accepted here, rejected there. We listen to conversations—one gland to another gland, one group of cells to another—discussing the distinctions of the material we have swallowed. "Can't fool us," we hear them saying.

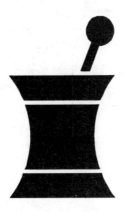

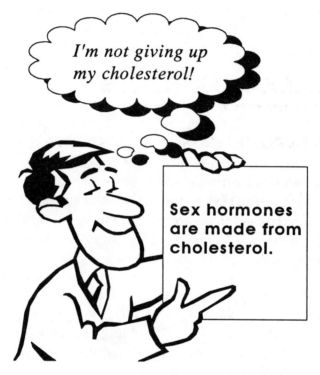

Reprinted from *New Facts About Fiber*
by Betty Kamen, Nutrition Encounter, Inc., 1991.

3

THE SEX HORMONES

TESTOSTERONE, ESTROGEN, PROGESTERONE

Testosterone, estrogen, and progesterone are hormones. More specifically, sex hormones. What? There are *three* sex hormones? In fact, there are several more, but these are the three principal sex hormones.

The word *testosterone* identifies a hormone made in the testes. But the word *estrogen* comes from the Greek, meaning "producing frenzy." It has been suggested that the difference in the sources of terminology reflects the bias of the male researchers who coined the term estrogen in 1927.[1]

We normally use the words testosterone and estrogen as if the two substances are male and female counterparts of each other. Actually, it's more complicated than that. Testosterone is one hormone of a general class of hormones called *androgens*. Androgens taken as a group, including testosterone, have the tissue-building and sex characteristics normally associated with the male sex hormone. *Estrogen*, like androgen, is the name for a class of hormones which includes several closely-related substances. So it's not really estrogen per se that produces many of the estrogen-related effects. When you read about estrogen and testosterone, understand that in the interest of clarity it's common to be a little loose with the jargon. To summarize: testosterone is only one of a broad class of hormones, the androgens. *Estrogen*, like *androgen* (but unlike *testosterone*), refers to an entire class of hormones. (See Figure 3 below.)

FIGURE 3

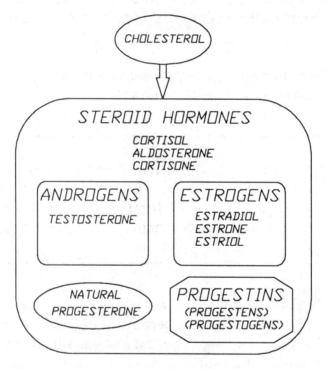

HOW CATEGORIES
OF STEROID HORMONES ARE RELATED

Estrogens, androgens, and natural progesterone are steroid hormones—all made from cholesterol. Keep in mind that even though progestins are referred to as steroids, they do not occur naturally in human physiology.

Confusion abounds surrounding the proper use of the term *progesterone*. As used here, *progesterone* or *natural progesterone* refers to one specific hormone—the one manufactured by your adrenal glands or ovaries. Progesterone is functionally related to, but *not* a member of, the class of hormones called *progestins*. Progestins may also be referred to as progestens, progestogens (also spelled progestegins in the medical literature), gestagens, or progestational agents. Confusing? Yes, but *all* progestins are synthetic hormones, or modifications of the natural hormone, closely resembling the hormone made in your body, but differing in significant ways.

The distinction between synthetic progestins and natural progesterone is extremely important.

Sometimes the term *progesterone treatment* is used to describe the therapeutic administration of a synthetic progestin rather than the real thing.

The difference between natural and synthetic progesterone is not unlike the difference between leather and vinyl car seats. They may look the same, but just wait till you get into the car on a hot day!

Progesterone is the primary building block for all the other steroid hormones. This alone distinguishes natural progesterone from synthetic progestins, which are incapable of performing this function. The one similarity between the synthetic and natural forms of progesterone is that they both promote endometrium secretion. Each can trigger uterine bleeding similar to menstrual flow, if needed.[2]

A natural hormone (found in humans or anywhere in nature) cannot be patented by a pharmaceutical company. A slight variation of the hormone, however, can be patented! Does this explain the popularity of synthetic hormones promoted by the drug companies? Would a board of directors allocate millions of dollars to develop a product for hormone therapy if it could not get patent protection for the substance involved?

FIGURE 4

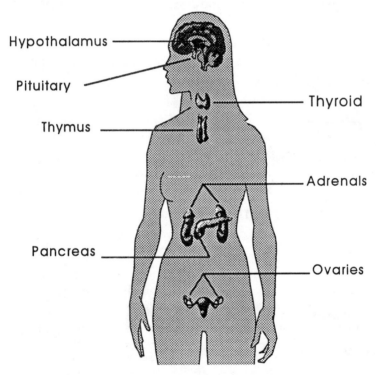

MAJOR HORMONE-PRODUCING GLANDS

Different types of hormone-secreting cells make up the endocrine system, which is influenced in part by the nervous system. Hormones are quite varied. The female and male sex hormones (estrogens and testosterone) are steroids.

BEHIND THE SCENES OF
HORMONE PRODUCTION

Before puberty, your adrenals—the pyramid-shaped glands that sit on top of each kidney—are responsible for manufacturing all the cholesterol-based, or steroid, sex hormones. (Your adrenal cortex is the part of each adrenal gland that actually makes the steroids.) Controlling this function is your pituitary, the tiny gland near the base of your brain—a gland so small it weighs no more than a paper clip.

Your pituitary, in turn, is regulated by your hypothalamus, the *master gland* which can almost be thought of as part of your brain. *This is the neurological link to steroid hormone production.* Messages from your brain are transmitted by way of your hypothalamus to your pituitary. Messenger hormones from your pituitary are then sent through your blood stream to your adrenal cortex, prompting the release of hormones that speed up or slow down the metabolic rate of cells throughout your body. So if you think of the adrenal cortex as a radio station broadcasting hormone signals to tissues, the pituitary can be thought of as the network hub that first sends the program (via a satellite link) to the affiliate station. And your hypothalamus—where the instructions originate—is like the production studio at the hub station.

In addition to sex-related hormones, your adrenal cortex manufactures the steroid hormones *cortisol* and *aldosterone*, among others.

Cortisol sounds like the more familiar *cortisone*, and in fact cortisone was one of the first adrenal steroids to be isolated and used medically. In large quantities it has the effect of reducing inflammation and suppressing immune responses.

But cortisol's primary function is to maintain adequate blood sugar levels. It does this by *stealing from protein and fat production* in order to support faster glucose production when needed. In your liver, this is accomplished by stimulating enzymes that prompt various amino acids to be used for making sugar rather than protein. In skeletal muscles, cortisol actually causes a transfer of amino acids out of the tissue and into the blood, where they travel to the liver to be made into glucose. Cortisol also contributes to the regulation of the day/night activity cycles and helps your body deal with stressful physiological situations in general. You can see how varied and sensitive hormone secretion can be in response to your environment.

Aldosterone is the hormone that controls potassium and magnesium excretion and sodium retention—processes designed to accommodate a time long past when diets were comprised of an abundance of potassium and magnesium and a shortage of sodium. Today, these metabolic functions appear to be backwards—contrary to our needs. The typical North American diet consists of far more sodium than potassium, throwing an important health-promoting ratio askew. Your body might be better served if your hormones and organs were more efficient at *retaining potassium* and *removing sodium*![3] Aldosterone is suppressed in the presence of potassium deficiency (or more typically, sodium excess).[4] Note the difference in the sodium and potassium ratios between processed and unprocessed foods in Table 1 on the next page.

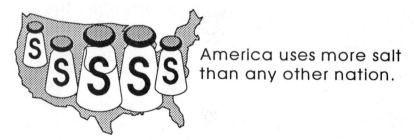

America uses more salt than any other nation.

TABLE 1
POTASSIUM & SODIUM CONTENT
OF INTACT & PROCESSED FOODS
in milligrams/100 grams food
(100 grams is approximately 3½ oz, or the
amount of food equal to the size of a closed fist)

	Potassium	Sodium
Flour, whole	360	3
White bread	100	540
Pork, uncooked	270	65
Bacon, uncooked	250	1400
Beef, uncooked	280	55
Corned beef	140	950
Haddock, uncooked	300	120
Haddock, smoked	190	790
Cabbage, uncooked	390	7
Cabbage, boiled	130	230
Horseradish, raw	564	8
Horseradish, prepared	290	96
Asparagus, raw	310	2
Asparagus, canned	250	200
Peas, fresh	380	1
Peas, frozen	135	115
Peas, canned	96	236
Peas, canned, served with ½ oz salted butter	99	374

Reprinted from *Everything You Always Wanted to Know About Potassium, But Were Too Tired to Ask,* Betty Kamen, Nutrition Encounter, Inc., 1992.

Aldosterone also affects fluid retention and blood pressure, partly to help keep sodium and potassium in balance.

Androgen production is the third and, for us, the most interesting product of the adrenal cortex.

Dehydroepiandrosterone, or DHEA (you can see why it is referred to by its initials), is the principal androgen made in the adrenals. Both testosterone and estradiol can be made from DHEA (recall that estradiol is an estrogen). In fact, before puberty DHEA is the major raw material for these hormones. This is important because testosterone and estradiol also have roles as growth hormones.

DHEA is available throughout your body. It is converted to stronger androgens, like testosterone, or subsequently to estradiol, as required. It's interesting to note that no testosterone is used by the brain—it's all made into an estrogen first. Keep this in mind if a male ever accuses you of not being able to "think like a man"!

At puberty, the male testes take over androgen production, far surpassing the production capacity of the adrenal cortex. This corresponds to the adolescent growth spurt occurring in boys, when skeletal muscles suddenly grow at a much greater rate under the influence of this new supply of male/growth hormones. The testes continue to produce androgens for life. We women, however, must rely on the adrenal cortex for androgenic hormones. Why do women need androgens at all? Primarily because of their tissue-building activity. Can you guess one reason why osteoporosis is more common in women than in men in this country?

As for women, estrogens and progesterone are produced by the ovaries between puberty and menopause. After menopause, the adrenal cortex is called on again to maintain the only supply of these vital hormones.

Flares from the hypothalamus and pituitary glands attempt to re-stimulate the ovaries into maintaining high estrogen levels at this time. *These bursts of control hormones are one source of hot flashes.* It's no surprise that your pituitary gland also has a role in controlling metabolism and body temperature.

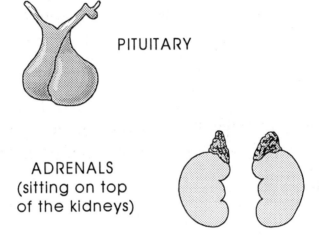

PITUITARY

ADRENALS
(sitting on top
of the kidneys)

What about progesterone? Figure 5 on page 42 shows the process (greatly simplified) by which your adrenal cortex manufactures steroid hormones. Starting with cholesterol (which can be stored to some extent in your adrenal gland, but should also be well supplied by your bloodstream), the first step is conversion to a substance called *pregnenolone.* Pregnenolone production normally limits the rate at which *all* the other steroid hormones can be created.[5]

The next maneuver is the construction of either progesterone or DHEA, and from there—through a number of other progressions that are not shown—the end result can be any one of a series of hormones.

FIGURE 5

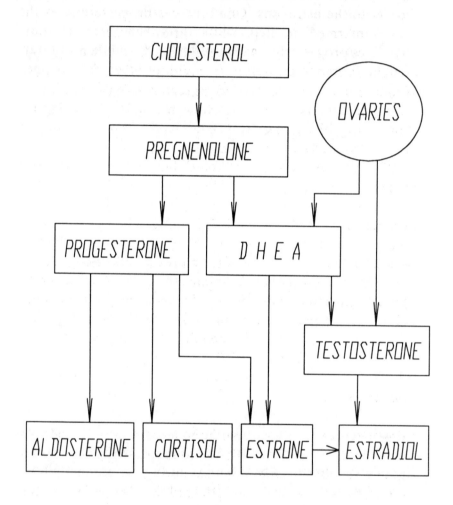

*PATHWAYS FROM CHOLESTEROL
TO SEX HORMONES*

This shows the chemical pathway from cholesterol to some important sex hormones that are synthesized in the adrenal cortex (simplified). Notice that there are several ways to make the estrogens *estrone* and *estradiol.*

There's something very significant about the pathways shown in Figure 5. As noted, there are two possible chemical routes to get to the estrogens. One involves progesterone as the main intermediate step, while the other chemical route bypasses progesterone and uses DHEA. So while progesterone is an important hormonal building block for estrogen production, it can be used to a greater or lesser extent for this purpose, depending on how much is available. It's something like going from one city to another using an interstate highway or getting there by traveling the back roads. You use a different route, but end up in the same place.

Progesterone is also manufactured in massive quantities by the placenta during pregnancy. The accelerated production starts in the fourth month and can reach 300 milligrams or more a day. This is 10 to 15 times the amount produced by your ovaries before pregnancy! If you have given birth to a child, remember the freedom from headaches and general feeling of well-being—even euphoria—that you felt as you entered your second trimester? High progesterone levels during pregnancy are believed to be responsible for the exhilaration.[6]

Progesterone levels vary with the menstrual cycle, and are considered to be closely linked to mood swings associated with PMS. *Estrogen dominance* during the second half of the cycle is the problem. Richard Kunin, M.D., of San Francisco, explains that estrogen and progesterone are in competition with each other at some receptor sites. In the presence of enough progesterone, estrogen is displaced, cancelling any effect that may be caused by too much estrogen. If progesterone levels are low, however, *estrogen dominates*. Even if *both* progesterone and estrogen are low, estrogen will be elevated.[7] And herein lies the trouble.

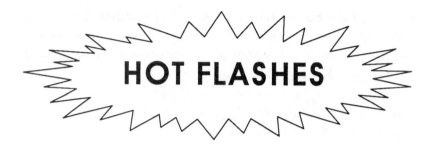

HOT FLASHES

➤ The only function that synthetic progestins and natural progesterone have in common is their ability to sustain human secretory endometrium.

Clinical Use of Sex Steroids, 1980[8]

➤ Synthetic progestins do not have the full spectrum of progesterone's biologic activity.

Clinical Use of Sex Steroids, 1980[9]

➤ Synthetic progestins have a wide variety of side effects.

Clinical Use of Sex Steroids, 1980[10]

➤ When oral progesterone is compared with medroxyprogesterone acetate (the most commonly prescribed progestin), the natural progesterone shows improved lipid profile, amenorrhea without endometrial problems, and no side effects.

Optimal Health Guidelines, 1992[11]

➤ Any change in the molecular configuration of steroids alters its effects.

Optimal Health Guidelines, 1992[12]

~~ ENDNOTES ~~ *The fantasy continues...*

We know we'll say goodbye to menstruation some day. Perhaps we already have.

There are memories, like the day of overflow when we wore our white skirt or white pants.

It's hard to imagine societies, even primitive ones, that did not have the use of sanitary napkins.

Whatever our *external* practices to catch the menstrual rivulet, very few of us really know the *inside* story. So back we go into ourselves in our fantasy, to watch in awe as estrogen and progesterone and other hormones fluctuate up and down, vying with each other for supremacy here, working in tandem there.

Ah! And now we see exactly why the chocolate cake we had for dinner interferes with the natural course of some of these events, and why PMS takes hold.

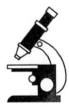

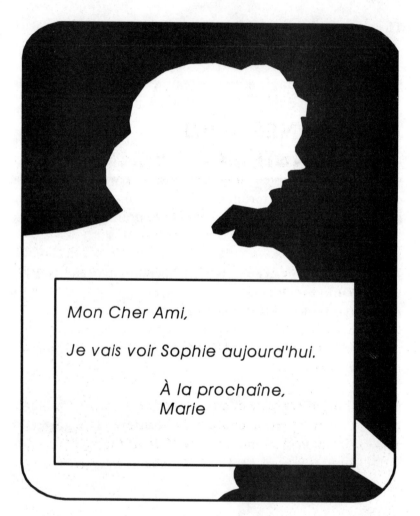

4

HORMONES AND
THE MENSTRUAL CYCLE

My friend Susan speaks for many women when she says,
"Menstruation makes me feel integrated, body and mind,
because it reminds me that I am *all* that I am—that what I
think and feel and want has much to do with what is going
on with me hormonally, nutritionally, and biochemically.
And it reminds me of this in a *good* way. Even if I do get a
little PMS, or a little crampy, it's fine because I take it as a
message that there's something imbalanced that needs my
attention."[1]

What a long way we've come! When I was a young teenager,
the word menstruation could only be uttered in whispers. If
you told your best friend that you "fell off the roof" (and you
would *only* tell your best friend), she knew that you were
menstruating.

Menstruation was known as "the poorlies" in nineteenth
century America, "the curse" in the twentieth century, and
in France you can still hear, "I'm going to see Sophie." But
the very oldest word for menstruation means "the woman's
friend."

Beth Richards, in *Blood of the Moon*, comments: "The simple fact that menstruation has evolved from 'woman's friend' to 'the curse' is a powerful symbol of the status of women."[2] *It may also be indicative of our declining health.*

As recently as 1970, Dr. Edgar Berman had PMS in mind when he declared that women weren't suitable for leadership positions because of their "raging hormonal influences." And as currently as 1993, the American Psychiatric Association concluded that women with severe PMS actually have a psychiatric disorder. In their current manual, PMS is cited under "mental disorders—not otherwise specified." If this arches your back, hear more: this group now wants to label the condition *"premenstrual dysphoric disorder"* (PMDD), to be listed as a specifically-defined psychiatric derangement under mood and depression.

How do you feel about a category of mental disorder that includes only women? The issue comes up for a vote as we go to press with this book. *Newsweek* comments: "Chances are there will be tears, irrationality and outbursts of anger—*elicited by neither hormones nor mental illness.*"[3]

Recently, the *Obstetrical and Gynecological Survey* stated that "PMS is probably a group of entities which includes various symptoms that occur during the 7 to 10 days before menstruation and disappear a few hours after the onset of menstruation." *Probably*? Isn't this the 1990s? Where have these researchers/physicians been? *Let's find out what really goes on.*

UNDERSTANDING MENSTRUATION

Figure 6 on page 50 shows the levels of estrogen and progesterone over a typical 28-day menstrual cycle. It also indicates a few of the control hormones produced by your pituitary.[4] In your effort to make decisions about hormone therapy, you may find it extremely beneficial to spend a few minutes with this chart.

Note that Day 1 represents the day that menstrual flow begins and that ovulation occurs at Day 14, stimulated by hormones. The 28-day cycle is average. A cycle that varies in both length and time of ovulation may not be abnormal— anything from a 20- to 40-day cycle could be considered okay.

> Women with irregular cycles and/or extended days of heavy flow, however, tend more toward the average 28-day cycle and normal flow after positive alterations in diet and lifestyle.

We'll start our narrative on Day 5 or so, when the menstrual flow subsides. This is the beginning of the pre-ovulatory, or *follicular* phase of the cycle, named for the follicles in your ovaries.

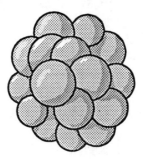

FIGURE 6

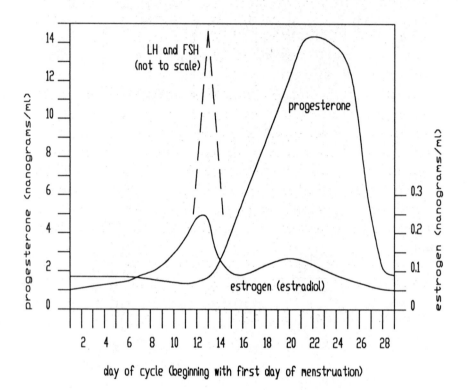

*TYPICAL PROGESTERONE
AND ESTROGEN LEVELS
DURING THE 28-DAY CYCLE*

Keep in mind that the concentrations of the two hormones are plotted on different scales. Where the curves cross, for example, there is 20 times more progesterone than estrogen circulating in the bloodstream.

Concentrations of progesterone and estrogen (estradiol) vary over the 28-day menstrual cycle. When progesterone peaks there should be about 140 times as much progesterone as estrogen.

FIGURE 7

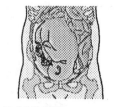

7,000,000 oocytes

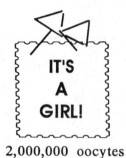

IT'S A GIRL!

2,000,000 oocytes

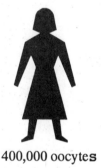

400,000 oocytes

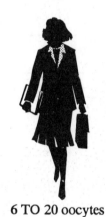

6 TO 20 oocytes

FOLLICLE REDUCTION RATE

When you reach puberty, each ovary contains about 400,000 follicles, down from about 7,000,000 after six months of embryonic life, and about 2,000,000 at birth. Each of these follicles contains an *oocyte* (each "o" is pronounced separately, so it's o-o-cyte). An oocyte is the human egg cell, the largest of all human cells. But only six to twenty of these begin to develop during a menstrual cycle, and only one continues to develop in only one ovary!

FIGURE 8

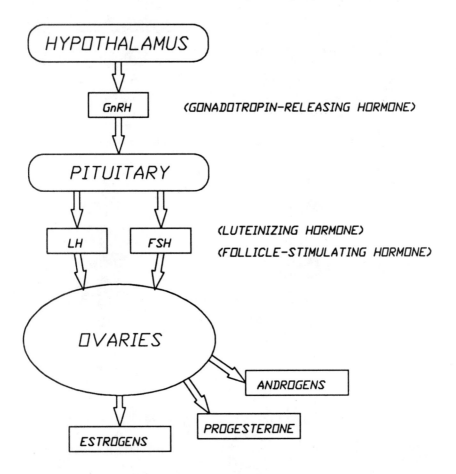

*LINKS BETWEEN THE BRAIN AND
SEX HORMONE PRODUCTION*

Chemical links between your brain and sex hormone production are complex. Your hypothalamus is partially controlled by nerve signals. It sends chemical messages to your pituitary, producing hormones that stimulate ovaries to go through various phases of ovulation and hormone production.

Development of the egg cell is sparked by the brain-controlled hypothalamus through a hormone called *gonadotropin-releasing hormone,* or GnRH. GnRH stimulates your pituitary to release two more substances into your blood stream: *luteinizing hormone* (LH) and *follicle-stimulating hormone* (FSH). These in turn act directly on your ovaries where they promote (1) the development and enlargement of the follicles and (2) the production of estrogen by the follicle cells. (See Figure 8 on page 52.)

The estrogen produced this way has an interesting effect. *It makes the follicles generate even more estrogen.* This is called a *positive feedback loop.* It's something like holding a microphone too close to a loudspeaker. Sound comes out of the speaker, is picked up by the microphone, gets amplified, and comes out of the speaker much louder—where it gets picked up again by the microphone. The result is an ear-splitting electronic whistle that doesn't go away until the volume is turned down or the microphone is turned off or covered.

Hormone interactions during the follicular phase of the menstrual cycle work in essentially the same way, except with the added complication of a *multiple* feedback loop. (See Figure 9 on page 54.) The estrogen produced by your ovaries surrounding the follicles tends to increase production in at least three different ways:

(1) by stimulating your hypothalamus to make more GnRH, which, in turn, stimulates your pituitary and ovaries
(2) by stimulating your pituitary to make more LH and FSH, which stimulates your ovaries
(3) by increasing the sensitivity of the cells surrounding the follicles in your ovaries to respond even *more* to the LH FSH from your pituitary.

FIGURE 9

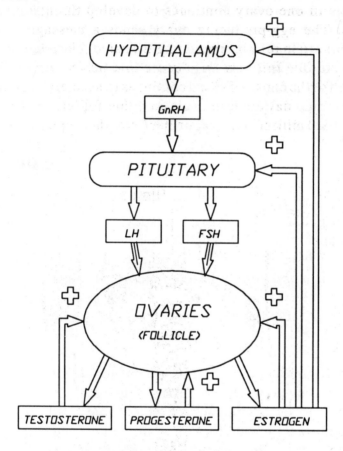

FOLLICULAR PHASE OF MENSTRUAL CYCLE,
BETWEEN MENSTRUATION AND OVULATION

Hormones produced by the ovarian follicles
have a positive feedback effect. More estrogen stimulates the hypothalamus to make more
GnRH, causing the pituitary to make more LH
and FSH, which stimulates the ovarian follicles
to produce even more estrogen. The plus signs
indicate the glands stimulated to produce more
hormones by the substances noted.

Follicles also communicate chemically with each other through a mechanism not yet fully understood. Only one follicle in one ovary continues to develop throughout the cycle. The egg-producing ovary sends a message to the other ovary to refrain from doing the same. *The presence of progesterone initiates this "cease and desist" order.* The growth of the chosen follicle continues to accelerate. During the last two days before ovulation, this follicle may be as large as 20 millimeters in diameter (over three-quarters of an inch!).

FIGURE 10

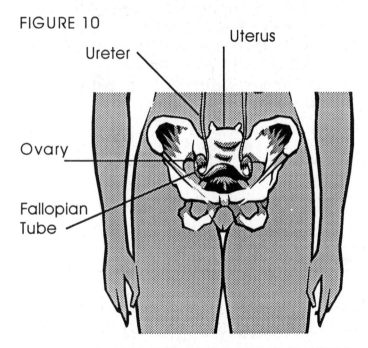

FEMALE REPRODUCTIVE SYSTEM

The ovary is 1¼ inches long. The uterus is a hollow muscular organ 3 inches long. The Fallopian tube is a 4½-inch tunnel to the uterus.

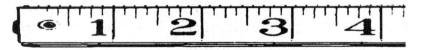

Progesterone is also responsible for increased female libido. This makes sense because of its associated production at the time of maximum fertility.

It is interesting to observe that in a certain island culture where yams containing progesterone precursors are a major staple of the local diet, libido is high but birth rate is relatively low. The ample supply of progesterone during the first half of the menstrual cycle may be responsible for reducing the rate of ovulation, while sex drive remains high throughout the month. (These people appear to be *extremely* happy!)

Back to business. On Day 14 of the cycle, LH and FSH swell to high levels, and this is known as the *pre-ovulatory surge.* The follicle moves to the wall of the ovary, enzymes degrade the ovary wall at the site of the protrusion, and the ovum is ejected from the follicle into your abdominal cavity. From there it finds its way to one of your Fallopian tubes for slow transportation to your uterus (and possible fertilization by a sperm on the way).

Don't think the follicle is done with its work. Immediately after release of the ovum on Day 14, the remaining cells continue to function. The follicle is now called the *corpus luteum,* and the post-ovulatory phase is called the *luteal phase* of the menstrual cycle. The corpus luteum is rich in cholesterol, conferring both its yellow color and its name. The word "luteal" means yellow.

FIGURE 11

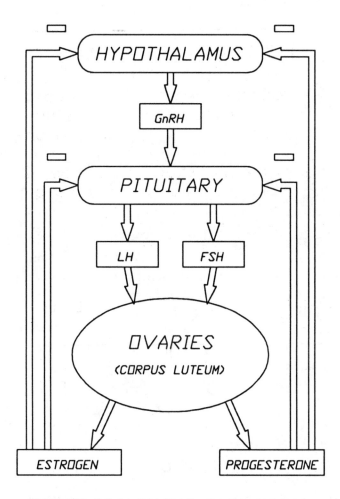

EVENTS FOLLOWING OVULATION

During the luteal phase, the feedback becomes negative. Estrogen and especially progesterone now inhibit the hypothalamus and pituitary from stimulating the ovaries into producing more hormones. The minus signs indicate suppression of glandular hormone production.

The follicle continues to produce estrogen, *but it also begins to manufacture a large amount of progesterone.* This grand flow of progesterone helps to suppress the development of other follicles so that only one follicle ejects an ovum. If, by chance, both of the ovaries have follicles that eject an ovum at almost exactly the same time —which happens about once every 300 periods—the result can be fraternal twins.

What about the runaway feedback loop? High levels of progesterone come to the rescue, shutting off the lofty rate of production of estrogen, GnRH, LH, and FSH. (See Figure 11 on page 57.) Circulating progesterone has an inhibiting effect on the production of GnRH by your hypothalamus and on the production of LH and FSH by your pituitary. The corpus luteum remains in your ovary and continues to grow for seven or eight days following ovulation. Then it degenerates, at which time the levels of progesterone and estrogen return to their initial levels.

During the luteal phase after ovulation, estrogen and progesterone stimulate growth and proliferation of the blood vessels and connective tissue in the wall of the uterus, ready to provide support and nutrients if a fertilized ovum is implanted.

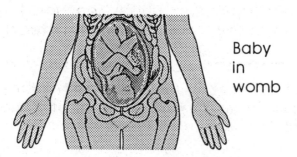

Baby
in
womb

If fertilization has not occurred about eight days after ovulation, this growth reverses, and your menstrual phase begins.

Prostaglandins (those produced by your uterus) stimulate the muscles within uterine walls, making them contract rhythmically and expel all the blood-rich and degenerating connective tissue from the inner surface of your uterine wall.

Throughout this process, the balance between estrogen and progesterone is critical. Maintaining an adequate level of progesterone appears to be particularly important—especially during the luteal phase when progesterone is keeping the positive feedback loop in check. The prostaglandins that contract your uterus can also cause contractions in other involuntary muscles. This is what causes menstrual cramps.

There is a tremendous amount to be learned in this area, but the evidence is beginning to point to a certain strategy for dealing with PMS.

Maintain your ability to produce progesterone and avoid external sources of estrogen (including beef loaded with estrogens from the animal's feed).

I believe that when progesterone and estrogen are in proper balance, premenstrual syndrome will be nothing more than words in a book.

¤

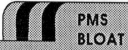

A Few Facts About PMS and Bloat

➤ Of course one should *never* drive and drink, but least of all just before your period! That's when you will show higher blood levels of alcohol. Premenstrual bloating probably accounts for this, since alcohol levels parallel those of body water. The lowest levels occur on the first day of menstrual bleeding.

➤ To reduce premenstrual bloating:

~ Balance your sodium/potassium intake. Additional information on how to do this is available in my book, *Everything You Always Wanted to Know About Potassium But Were Too Tired to Ask.*[5]

~ Add natural progesterone to your daily regime. (See suggestions later in this book.)

~ Don't use Stimerol chewing gum. It contains glycyrrhizinic acid, a main component of licorice, which can induce sodium retention.[6]

MEMOS **PMS BLOAT**

➤ The increased levels of sex steroids that occur during a normal menstrual cycle affect the rate of caffeine elimination. Clearance of caffeine is slower in the luteal phase.[7]

➤ Vascular congestion may contribute to water retention. Sexual activity relieves such congestion.[8]

➤ Natural herbal diuretics include raspberry leaf, marjoram, and thyme teas, available at your local health store. These herbs do not have the deleterious effects of prescription diuretics.[9]

➤ Vitamin B_6 is especially valuable in reducing premenstrual edema.[10]

➤ Drugs that function as diuretics can have very serious side effects. Using such diuretics requires close medical supervision with regular blood tests to check body salt balance. Overuse of diuretics can upset your potassium and sodium levels, which can make your PMS worse.[11]

MEMOS

CAUSES FOR PMS

➤ Possible causative factors of PMS:
- ~ progesterone deficiency
- ~ estrogen/progesterone imbalance
- ~ thyroid hypofunction
- ~ antidiuretic hormone excess
- ~ fluid retention
- ~ shifting endorphin levels
- ~ serotonin alterations
- ~ abnormal prostaglandin action
- ~ vitamin deficiency (especially B_6)
- ~ ovarian infection
- ~ yeast overgrowth
- ~ hypoglycemia

Obstetrical and Gynecological Survey, 1990[12]
Journal of Nurse-Midwifery, 1990[13]
Journal of Reproductive Medicine, 1990[14]

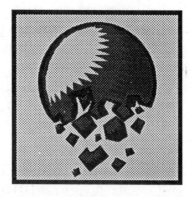

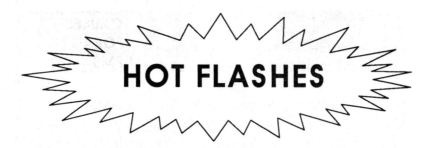

HOT FLASHES

➤ Lack of ovulation is common in those involved in intensive athletic activity without supplemental support.
Pediatric Clinics of North America, 1989[15]

➤ Lack of ovulation is common in those who limit food intake excessively and do not include nutrient supplementation.
Pediatric Clinics of North America, 1989[16]

➤ Food choices are often responsive to the hormonal changes in your menstrual cycle.
American Journal of Clinical Nutrition, 1993[17]

➤ The consumption of foods and beverages which are high in sugar content is associated with the prevalence of PMS.
Journal of Reproductive Medicine, 1991[18]

➤ Women with PMS might have disturbances of their hypothalamus and adrenal glands.
Journal of Clinical Endocrinology and Metabolism, 1990[19]

➤ Caloric intake increases under the progesterone curve during the luteal phase.
Fertility and Sterility, 1988[20]

➤ Free radicals (runaway cells caused by toxins or rancidity, as found in salad dressings and other processed foods) may play a role in the regression of the corpus luteum.

Journal of Reproduction and Fertility, 1992[21]

➤ Many women report that eliminating coffee, tea, caffeinated colas, and chocolate relieves PMS breast tenderness.

Anecdotal, 1993

➤ Menstrual problems including amenorrhea (lack of menstruation), irregular cycles, or abnormal uterine bleeding represent 50 percent of adolescents' gynecologic complaints.

Hormone Research, 1991[22]

➤ Amenorrhea may be a sign of late puberty or of a problem affecting the hypothalamus, the pituitary, or the ovaries.

Hormone Research, 1991[23]

~~~

"Mom is yelling again.
It must be that time of month."

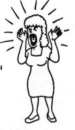

  "I must have some ice cream;
It must be that time of month."

IT DOESN'T HAVE TO BE THIS WAY!

~~ ENDNOTES ~~ *The fantasy continues...*

The decades progess and we note how much more slowly repair cells move as they head toward a scratch, how diminished in number they are for its mending, how much longer it takes for replacement cells to reach your suntanned skin. Note how the bountiful supply of organ reserve—granted with such generosity to youth—abates.

See the negative effects of toxins—their cells victorious in battle with immune cells. See the benefits of antioxidants—hopefully, the victors. Watch as mushed and mangled foods produce warriors—fighting the wrong cause. Watch the nutrient-dense foods provide ammunition for triumph. Note that more of the good guys are required today than yesterday—because we are one day older.

Can we learn from experience? Will we acknowledge today that we will need even *more* tomorrow because we will be yet another day older?

Aging—it takes us by surprise. Our ovaries put up a sign: *Out of Business.* Nature seems to be saying, "We don't need any more like you." *Not to worry*: nature doesn't want us to go without. *Another organ gets pressed into service.*

We observe that wrinkling occurs more rapidly in one woman than another, the same age. The fantasy demonstrates exactly *how* and *why* aging changes take place at menopause. We note that a menopausal woman *can* continue to manufacture hormones—just the right amount to maintain optimal health, including healthy bones and a healthy sex life. But the message appears to be:

Now we need a little more help.

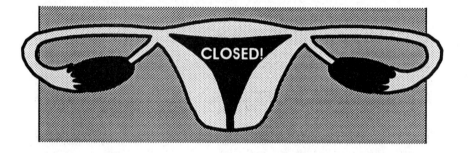

5

HORMONES AND MENOPAUSE

IT'S NOT ALL BAD NEWS

Happy 50th birthday! If you are an average American woman celebrating a half century of life, chances are your varicose veins and your belly stick out, your dimples and breasts sag, and you sport a bigger nose and droopier earlobes than ever before. (Too bad your vision is so good!) Your doctor, however, is concerned about a transformation that your mirror does not directly reflect: *the shutdown of estrogen production.* Happy birthday?

Actually, the processes leading to these aging overtures began decades before this landmark year. Various parts of your skeleton, for example, start their downslide when you are in your twenties. You can be sure there has been a constant reduction of the mechanical properties of your bone with age—even if tests which your physician may have administered show no loss of bone density until you approach menopause.[1] (An inexpensive test using *photons*, which are no more than beams of very high-intensity light, can now positively define the status of your bone density with 95 percent accuracy.)

The output of very important hormones start their plunge in your thirties. In fact, in some ways you begin to age from the moment you are born.

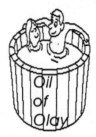

You can bathe in Oil of Olay forever, but you will get old—if that is all you use in your attempt to delay the visual impact of the aging process!

The news, however, is not totally negative. As Hallmark cards inform us, *Fifty Can Be Nifty.* Your adrenal glands pump estrogens even as your ovaries curtail their manufacture. Although adrenal estrogen is not as powerful as ovarian estrogen, your body is most appreciative for the offering. Called *estrone,* this contribution is converted from weak male hormones in your fat cells. The healthier your adrenals, the less apt you are to suffer common menopausal complaints—depression, sweating, vaginal dryness, and that dynamic devilish duo, *hot flashes and wakeful nights.*

Significantly more fatty tissue is concentrated just below the abdominal skin of perimenopausal women (the stage prior to menopause).[2] The tendency for women in their forties to experience "middle-age spread" may not be without purpose or benefit. Heavier women have the least severe osteoporotic symptoms. Don't get too excited about the benefits of overweight, however; *the estrogenic hormone level is usually more out of balance in those who are overweight, especially in the presence of progesterone deficiency.*

Menstrual cycles often become irregular as you approach menopause. Even when you do menstruate, you do not ovulate—despite normal estrogen levels.

> Without the cyclic increase and fall in progesterone during the perimenopausal stage, endometrial shedding is not triggered in a timely fashion. So menstrual cycles become irregular.

Carpal tunnel syndrome is one disorder which tends to increase with menopause, resulting in pain and burning or tingling in the fingers and hand, sometimes extending to the elbow. Caused by the compression of a nerve, it has been known for a decade that carpal tunnel syndrome is linked to vitamin B_6 (pyridoxine) deficiency.[3] Vitamin B_6 in supplemental form, therefore, may be helpful. According to a report published in the *Annals of the New York Academy of Sciences*, 1990, vitamin B_6 is safe at doses of 100 milligrams a day.[4] The addition of a daily dose of magnesium (400 milligrams) along with the vitamin B_6 (50 milligrams) increases the benefit. It could take about 2 to 12 weeks for this remedy to work. Although carpal tunnel syndrome is common among both male and female computer keyboard users, hormonal changes at menopause appear to exacerbate the condition for women.[5]

Now let's dispel a few menopause myths.

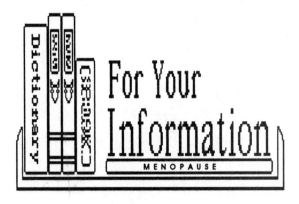

For Your Information

MENOPAUSE

WHAT MENOPAUSE WON'T DO

➢ Menopause itself does not cause significant weight gain. No serious differences are found between pre- and postmenopausal women with regard to total body weight, body mass index, waist-hip ratio, and *total* abdominal fat tissue areas.

International Journal of Obesity, 1992[6]

➢ Popular medical view to the contrary, natural menopause does not have negative mental health consequences for the majority of middle-aged healthy women.

Journal of Consulting and Clinical Psychology, 1990[7]

WHAT MENOPAUSE WILL DO

➢ Blood pressure increases with age—or, more accurately, as a result of aging in people living the usual Western lifestyle with its destructive dietary habits. *Ovarian failure appears to be protective against this increase.*

American Journal of Epidemiology, 1989[8]

➢ Estradiol, a form of estrogen, enhances vulnerability to schizophrenia, but *the effect is lowered again during menopause.*

European Archives of Psychiatry and Clinical Neuroscience, 1991[9]

➢ Menopause brings with it a total freedom from pregnancy concern, and, for many, a new level of sexual enjoyment along with this freedom.

Healthy menopausal women the world over

MISCELLANEOUS MENOPAUSE FACTS

➤ A woman in the United States can now expect to live for thirty years or more past menopause in what the medical journals refer to as a "state of estrogen deprivation."
Drug Intelligence and Clinical Pharmacy, 1988[10]

➤ The earlier the menopause, the greater the need to improve lifestyle or seek the right kind of treatment.
Union Medicale du Canada, 1992[11]

➤ Bone loss related to menopause begins during the irregular menstruation period before menopause.
Calcified Tissue International, 1991[12]

➤ Regular sexual activity is beneficial in maintaining a healthy, functional vagina.
Postgraduate Medicine, 1992[13]

➤ High intake of dietary fiber, vitamin C, and beta-carotene decrease the risk for postmenopausal breast cancer.
International Journal of Cancer, 1991[14]

➤ The time between menopause and the occurrence of hip fractures averages about 30 years. (Some physicians place this number at 10 or 15 years.)
Lancet, 1993[15]

➤ Osteoporosis begins several years prior to menopause, *before any decrease in estrogen levels.*
Canadian Journal of Obstetrics and Gynecology, 1991[16]

Note something very interesting about this last fact: *Osteoporosis begins several years before menopause, yet estrogen levels are normal up to the time of menopause.* More about this later!

AGE AT MENOPAUSE

At the turn of the century, the average menopausal woman in this country was about 45. Today, the average age of the *climactic*, as it is called in the medical literature, is closer to 50 or 51.

> For reasons not understood, age at menopause is significantly earlier among left-handed women than those who are right-handed.[17]

Active smokers experience menopause 1.7 years sooner than non-smokers. The typical age of onset in nonsmokers is 49.8; in passive smokers (nonsmokers who live or work with smokers), it's 49.1; and in active smokers, 48.13 years. These differences depend on the duration of smoking—increasing with the number of smoked cigarettes to as much as 2.4 years in smokers of greater than 20 cigarettes per day and to 3 years if your mother was also a smoker.[18]

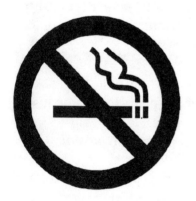

Evidence suggests that cigarette smoking has an anti-estrogenic effect in women.[19]

HOT FLASHES

Too many studies explore disease rather than health. A group of investigators reporting in *Lancet*, 1992, broke from this tradition when they examined Japanese women among whom hot flashes are infrequent. They found a very high intake of *phyto-estrogen*s (100- to 1,000-fold more than in American women), along with other foods which have some estrogen activity.

Phyto-estrogens are associated with these soy products:
- tofu
- miso
- aburage
- atuage
- koridofu
- soybeans
- boiled beans

Estrogenic activity of phyto-estrogens may help to explain why hot flashes are not as common among these women.[20] They occupy the same receptor sites as estrogen, so they help to prevent excess estrogen from "taking hold" thereby preventing estrogen overload. Other phyto-estrogens are black cohosh, alfalfa, licorice, and pomegranates.

Women have reported that they have fewer and less intense hot flashes when they have a fever. The reasons? Perhaps the following:

(1) Because of competing heat-regulatory drives, the characteristic changes do not occur. The temperature inhibits whatever it is that launches the hot flash.

(2) Some product of the fever process masks the changes that occur during hot flashes.[21]

We don't need double-blind, controlled studies to tell us that those who experience hot flashes during the night tend to sleep less efficiently. But it sure is hopeful to know that such information is cited in the medical literature, as in the journal, *Sleep*.[22] It's an indication that the professionals are finally paying attention.

Vitamin E has a stabilizing effect on estrogen levels, so supplementation with this fat-soluble nutrient may increase hormone production in those who are vitamin E-deficient.

The increased hormone production caused by supplemental vitamin E helps to reduce hot flashes. Vitamin C and bioflavonoids have also been demonstrated to be helpful in minimizing hot flashes.

Many questions about hot flashes remain unanswered. According to the *New York Academy of Sciences,* the flashes may start much earlier and continue far longer than is commonly recognized by physicians or acknowledged in textbooks of gynecology. Hot flashes are not static; patterns may change with time. For some women, they become less frequent and less intense; for others, they may continue at hourly intervals well into old age.[23]

IT DOESN'T HAVE TO BE THAT WAY!

¤

MEMOS

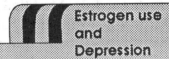
Estrogen use and Depression

Antidepressant Effects of Estrogen Therapy

ABSTRACT: The potential antidepressant effects of estrogen replacement therapy were examined cross-sectionally in a population of 1190 women 50 years and older living in Rancho Bernardo, California. Of the total, 294 (24.7pecent) were currently using estrogen. Among women aged 50-59 years, those currently using estrogen replacement therapy had a significantly higher rate of Beck Depression Inventory scores of 13 or higher than all untreated women of the same age and *they had higher average depressive symptom scores than women who had never used estrogen.*

Source: Palinkas LA; Barrett-Connor E. Estrogen use and depressive symptoms in postmenopausal women. *Obstetrics and Gynecology*, 1992 Jul, 80(1):30-6.

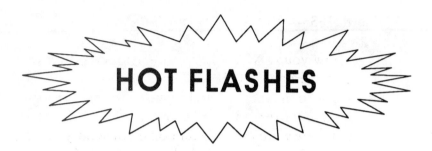

HOT FLASHES

➤ Only five percent of women receiving hormone therapy said they had requested the therapy from their practitioner.
British Journal of General Practice, 1991[24]

➤ Sixty-one percent of women receiving hormone therapy said they obtained information about hormone replacement therapy from either television, magazines, or newspapers—not from their physicians.
British Journal of General Practice, 1991[25]

➤ Certain steroid hormones are found in lesser quantities in women who experience early menopause than in late menopausal women.
Journal of the Medical Association of Thailand, 1992[26]

➤ Glucose and cholesterol values are significantly higher in postmenopausal women.
International Journal of Obesity, 1992[27]

➤ Eighty percent of women on replacement therapy say they would have liked more information about menopause before its onset.
British Journal of General Practice, 1991[28]

~~ ENDNOTES ~~ *The fantasy continues...*

No matter how young we are in spirit, our physical appearance reflects the aging process—especially when our fantasy escorts us to the internal architecture of our *bones*. We can see the *disequilibrium* between normal bone formation and bone loss. We watch as our skeleton is constantly "doing and undoing." We see its changing density. Not much happens to size or shape—only to *porosity*. A panorama of years helps us to observe osteoporosis setting in—a wooden rod replacing one of steel.

In our fantasy, science is advanced enough to understand the dynamics. We see *how* bone changes as it heals, shapes, and grows. We catch the magic of *how* calcium gets incorporated, *how* cartilage hardens, *how* vitamin C affects collagen. We see one kind of cell looking for old bone to dissolve: *Pacman wiping out its victims*. We follow with awe as another kind of cell gives birth to new bone: *the miracle of creation*.

Even at age 90, we note that one can still mend bone in the presence of bone-building tools. Now we know that bone is not unchanging, but forever shifting—young or old. We see that the factors that make all this happen efficiently are dependent on individual life choices. We note how different it is when the appropriate nutrients are present. *We see that bone loss may be a natural accompaniment of aging, but that it need not have adverse implications.*

We look at an older woman, and because this is fantasy we see her go back in time to childhood and watch the aging process in reverse. As she grows younger, we see larger eyes, shorter nose, smoother skin, and fuller cheeks. We see bones so rubbery and supple they do not break when she falls.

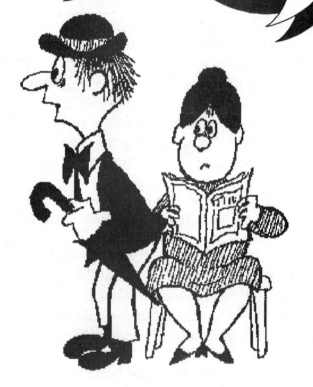

6

ABOUT BONE

Bone is far more complicated than you might imagine. It's essentially a composite of two types of material: tendon-like organic collagen and hard inorganic calcium phosphate crystals. The combination can be likened to fiberglass, which is comprised of both flexible cloth and brittle plastic resin. Together, they make a consolidated structure that's strong and tough. Flexible, spongy collagen would be useless by itself in bone, just as the brittle calcium phosphate would fracture much too easily on its own. But they combine to make an amazingly strong and resilient structure.

Too often, environmental factors interact to prevent full expression of your genotype—your inherited bone-density potential.[1] According to studies reported in *Osteoporosis International*, 1990, twenty-three percent of bone variability can be attributed to habits from infancy to the present.[2] These variations include:
> food choices
> sports activities
> combination of foods eaten at one meal
> frequency of dieting
> skipping meals

For females, bone mass accumulation by age twenty is also associated with maternal bone mass.

Hereditary contributions from your mother play an overwhelmingly critical role in your bone health.

But nature is forgiving; good environmental influences on bone consolidation during the decades before menopause may be more important in promoting optimal or peak bone mass, thereby helping to prevent or delay the postmenopausal onset of osteoporotic fractures.[3]

Until the time of menopause, bone mass is also enhanced by child-bearing and lactation; beyond menopause, environmental factors dominate.[4]

If you are an average healthy adult, you lose 500 milligrams of calcium from your bones every day.[5] That's half a gram! At that rate, your bones would be reduced to powder in just a few years. What saves your skeleton is the fact that 500 milligrams of calcium are deposited *back* into your bone structure daily. Special bone cells called *osteoblasts* take calcium and phosphorus from your blood and deposit crystals in your bone structure. But other cells, *osteoclasts*, remove those same crystals and return calcium and phosphorus to your blood plasma. The outer layer of your bones—the calcium phosphate—is the material subject to the actions of these cells. This is very convenient—it makes the calcium readily accessible when needed.

Why this seemingly risky interchange of bone material *into* and *out of* your bones? *Because it's extremely important for your body to preserve a specific concentration of calcium in your blood plasma.*

The precise level of calcium is maintained even at the expense of the structural integrity of your bones. You see, calcium is also responsible for:

> ➤ nerve cell communication
> ➤ contraction of muscle cells
> ➤ blood-clotting efficiency
> ➤ the function of very important enzymes
> ➤ the production of certain proteins

FIGURE 12

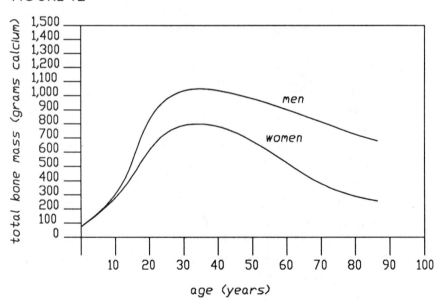

RELATIONSHIP BETWEEN AGE AND BONE MASS

Men suffer from osteoporosis too, but, in this country, the loss of bone mass is far more severe in women.

Your total blood calcium must be very carefully maintained at about 10 milligrams per 100 milliliters of plasma (about a quarter of a gram in an average adult woman). But calcium is continually being filtered out by your kidneys and excreted. To maintain the precise balance, bone tissue is a natural place to store and retrieve calcium as required.

Since calcium appears to abound in food, why can't you get enough of this mineral for bone health from your dinner plate? *Because dietary calcium is unreliable*:

> At best, intestinal absorption of calcium supplied by food is never more than about 50 percent efficient.

> An excess of fat reduces calcium absorption.[6]

> Calcium absorption decreases with age. The decline starts earlier for women.[7]

> Antacids, tetracyclines, laxatives, diuretics, and other drugs impede calcium absorption.[8]

> Individual differences result in extreme variations. For example, studying the calcium retention of two normal five-year-olds eating the same food showed that one retained 78 percent more calcium than the other![9] *We are not all the same.*

> There is a direct correlation between salt intake and calcium excretion.

Phosphorus metabolism is driven by the same hormones that control calcium. This makes sense, considering the fact that calcium and phosphorus are incorporated together into bone structure. But this assumes a ratio of calcium and phosphorus that would be found in a natural diet. All too often, just as with sodium and potassium, we subject ourselves to an *unbalanced* ratio. The main reason is the excess phosphorus we consume with our sodas, meat products, cheese, baked goods, and other highly-processed foods. *Too much phosphorus prevents the proper assimilation of new calcium into your bone tissue.* An additional problem? Phosphorus levels are not as tightly controlled as calcium levels!

¤

MEMOS

BONE

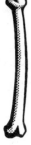
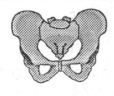
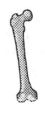

Bone is a specialized connective tissue that, together with cartilage, makes up the skeleton.

These tissues serve three functions. They are:

(a) a mechanical support and site of muscle attachment for locomotion,

(b) protection for vital organs and bone marrow, and

(c) a metabolic reserve of ions for the entire organism, especially calcium and phosphorus.

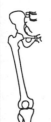
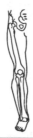
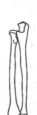
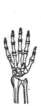
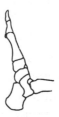

FIGURE 13

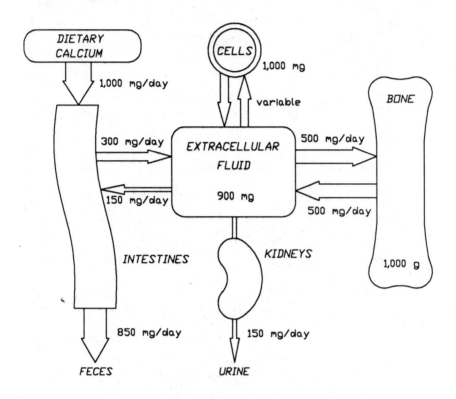

CALCIUM: IN AND OUT OF BONE

This represents the typical daily flow of calcium in and out of bone tissue. Less than a third of dietary calcium is absorbed.

FIGURE 14

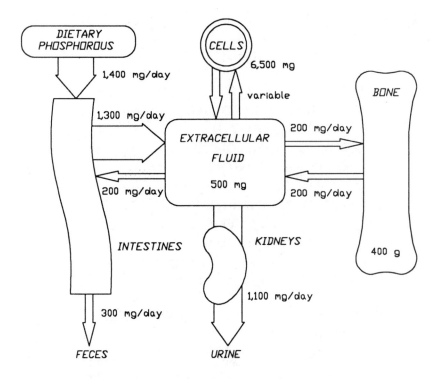

PHOSPHORUS: IN AND OUT OF BONE

This represents the typical daily flow of phosphorus in and out of bone tissue. Absorption is above 90 percent. Excessive dietary phosphorus can interfere with proper utilization of calcium.

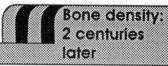

Bone density:
2 centuries
later

LEARNING ABOUT BONE DENSITY FROM COFFINS IN ENGLISH BURIAL CRYPTS

The incidence of osteoporotic hip fractures has been increasing faster than the rate expected if it were adjusted for life expectancy. The recent restoration of a London church, during which bone fragments dating from 1729 to 1852 were recovered, provided a novel opportunity to compare the occurrence of historical bone loss with that of present-day women.

The rate of bone loss is significantly greater today than in women from two centuries ago, both pre- and postmenopausally. The researchers saw the typical decline in premenopausal bone density in present-day women but found no significant loss in these preserved samples. This suggests that a 70-year-old woman today would have a lower bone density than a 70-year-old woman who had lived two centuries ago.

Lancet, 1993[10]

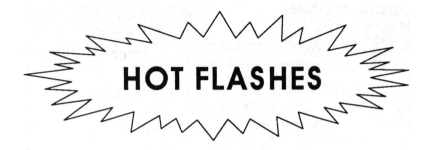

HOT FLASHES

➤ Low hip-bone density is a stronger predictor of hip fracture than bone density at other sites.
   Lancet, 1993[11]

➤ The more caffeine, the more bone loss.
   Calcified Tissue International, 1992[12]

➤ The development of optimal bone mass early in life is more effective in preventing osteoporosis than traditional measures used later in life.
   Clinical Rheumatology, 1989; *Osteoporosis International*, 1990[13,14]

➤ After menopause, environmental factors override the advantages of reproductive and breastfeeding history for bone mineral density.
   American Journal of Epidemiology, 1992[15]

➤ After age 30 to 35, the total amount of bone shrinks about 10 percent per decade in women.
   Geriatrics, 1974[16]

➤ After age 30 to 35, the total amount of bone shrinks about 5 percent per decade in men.
   Geriatrics, 1974[17]

➤ Women over 55 and men over the age of 60 have had enough bone loss to produce at least one break.
Geriatrics, 1974[18]

➤ White women of small stature are at greatest risk for osteoporosis.
Startling New Facts About Osteoporosis, 1992[19]

➤ The reduction of bone mass with age is significantly greater in alcoholics, especially after age sixty.
Clinical Orthopedics and Related Research, 1973[20]

➤ *Any* dysfunction of *any* regulatory system leads to changes in bone formation or resorption, and ultimately to skeletal disease.
British Dental Journal, 1992[21]

➤ Cadmium concentrations in Pecos Indian bones were 50 times lower than those of contemporary humans.
Environmental Health Perspectives, 1991[22]

➤ The percentage of total body lead found in bones can range from 78 percent at age 20 to 96 percent at age 80, placing a burden on the body's bone health as we age.
Environmental Research, 1990[23]

➤ The osteoblasts can't make new bone unless the osteoclasts have done their work to provide the necessary space.
Optimal Health Guidelines, 1990[24]

~~ ENDNOTES ~~ *The fantasy continues...*

Back in our fantasy, we see exchanges taking place between our bones and blood in such great quantity that their number could dwarf the total transactions made on the floor of the stock market on its busiest day. Instead of brokers directing the responses, hormones are at the helm.

We see the hormones moving calcium into our blood from two places—our intestines and our bones. We jump back quickly to get out of the way of the darting messages sent to these two warehouses—signals to release their calcium inventory into our blood. We observe the more important aspects—those that influence calcium's deposition, storage, transportation, and arrival at key locations. We are impressed by the complicated internal traffic control manipulated by the hormones.

And then we see that it's not just estrogen that regulates these transactions. This private network is dependent on more than just one hormone.

Even more fascinating, we see that the constant inflow and outflow of bone materials also allows for bone modification in response to our individual changing requirements. It allows for our bones to thicken and strengthen when we exercise regularly and to heal after they break. Now we know that bone is living tissue, that bones can be compressed with surprising, maybe even *alarming*, facility.

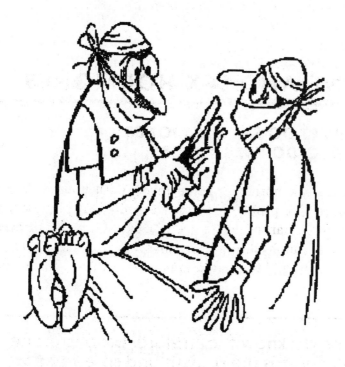

"It's going to rain. I can feel it in her bones."

Reprinted from *Startling New Facts About Osteoporosis* by Betty Kamen, Nutrition Encounter, Inc., 1992

7

BONE AND SEX HORMONES

SO WHAT DO SEX HORMONES HAVE TO DO WITH BONES?

What do sex hormones have to do with bones? A good question! The problem is that we don't really know more than a small part of the answer. "Key ingredients of osteoporosis pathophysiology are missing from the prevailing understanding,"[1] to use the language of the technical journals.

We do know that natural progesterone stimulates the growth and spread of osteoblasts,[2] and that other sex steroid levels play a role in the physiology of bone![3]

In more general terms, we know that serious loss of bone mass is closely correlated with menopause. During the first six years following its onset, the decrease in mineral density of some bones is *three to ten times higher than the change in the decade prior to menopause.*[4] And the biggest change in menopause is the decline of estrogens and progesterone!

So it has been logical to assume that artificially replacing the lost hormones could have a beneficial effect on bone strength.

In fact it does—sort of. Synthetic estrogen, used as estrogen replacement therapy (abbreviated *ERT*, or more recently, *HRT* for hormone replacement therapy), does in fact reduce the rate of bone loss.[5] It also decreases the incidence of bone fractures by 50 percent, as demonstrated when comparing groups of postmenopausal women who do not receive ERT.[6] If this is so, why is controversy so prevalent?

For starters, not every researcher gets the same result. In one extensive study spanning 14 years, no decrease in hip fractures at all could be detected with the use of ERT.[7] But let's allow the benefit of doubt and assume that fractures really can be reduced by 50 percent. This would be a compelling statistic, but it would still be 50 percent too much.

If the dilemma of osteoporosis were being addressed effectively, there would be almost *no* fractures! Aside from a rare accident, older women simply do not subject their bones to stresses that should cause them to break. Twisting your foot the wrong way as you step down a curb should not cause a fracture! And how many skydiving senior citizens do you know?

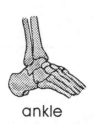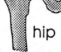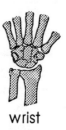

ankle   hip   wrist

Common breaking points

Currently, there are 1,500,000 fractures every year attributable to osteoporosis.[8]

Even if we could treat all the women who might benefit —reducing the number of fractures to 750,000—we'd still have a big problem. And the number of women aged 65 and older is expected to double by the year 2000![9]

According to a recent report by the Study of Osteoporotic Fractures Research Group (a combined effort of several major university hospitals including more than 8,000 women, reported in *Lancet,* 1993), *the decline in bone density with age does not entirely account for the increasing risk of hip fractures with aging.* Environmental exposures play a large role! We are more or less putting all our eggs in one basket when we focus almost entirely on sex-hormone decreases as a causative factor for broken bones.[10]

Here's another intriguing fact: tamoxifen is an anti-estrogen drug given to breast-cancer prone women to block the uptake of estrogen hormones. If lack of estrogen is the cause of osteoporosis, one would expect that tamoxifen would cause loss of bone density. But according to the *New England Journal of Medicine,* 1992, tamoxifen does no such thing![11]

Decreased hormonal output is not the only cause of bone density loss, and this loss is not the only cause of broken bones. Lower hormonal production is, however, a significant contributing factor.

A 1992 report in the *Southern Medical Journal* concludes that *osteoporosis is a preventable and treatable condition.*

¤

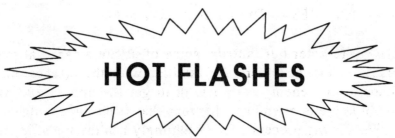

HOT FLASHES

➢ Osteoporotic fractures have an enormous impact on mortality, productivity, independence, and self-esteem.
Southern Medical Journal, 1992[12]

➢ Adult women face a 15-percent lifetime risk of a hip fracture, the annual cost of which is estimated at $7.3 billion in the United States.
Osteoporosis International, 1992[13]

➢ People with chronic bronchitis treated with corticosteroids, even at low doses, are at risk for osteoporosis.
Osteoporosis International, 1992[14]

➢ Bone loss can be caused by *acidosis*. Acidosis occurs for many reasons, including poor breathing (as in bronchitis).
John Lee, M.D., 1993[15]

➢ Major risk factors for osteoporosis include age, initial bone density, and calcium absorption.
Wiener Medizinische Wochenschrift, 1990[16]

➢ The rate of broken bones has been increasing in the female population twice as fast as population growth.
Geriatrics, 1974[17]

~~ ENDNOTES ~~ *The fantasy continues...*

As we re-enter our fantasy, some of us are amazed at the ongoing battle. Others are familiar with the clashes and know about enemy cells trying to get the upper hand as immune cells attempt to prevent that from happening—a never-ending process in our seemingly healthy body. Most of us know that cells carrying seeds of damage can be overpowered and attacked by immune cells with killer status, but we had no idea how frequently it happens—that it is so much a part of everyday life!

The ending is not always a happy one. The corrupt cell can split, unchallenged, and become two, then four, then eight. When proliferation is out of control, we call it *cancer.*

Sometimes we invite the trouble. ("We have met the enemy and it is us.") We watch as *synthetic* hormones attempt to play real-life roles. (There goes the neighborhood.) Try as they will, they cannot imitate. No Oscar Award here—*the performance of the look-alike stuff just isn't good enough.*

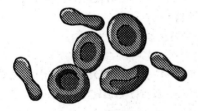

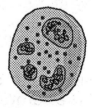

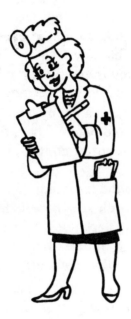

Your index finger on your left hand shows no sign of osteoporosis. Now I'm going to refer you to a colleague who will examine the index finger on your right hand.

8

SEX HORMONES AND CANCER AND OTHER SIDE EFFECTS

WHAT ABOUT SEX HORMONES AND CANCER?

Then there's the cancer risk. Perhaps more than any other disease, we have come to regard cancer as the Grim Reaper of our time. But the process that makes a cell cancerous is the same process by which a cell grows, replicates, and propagates itself. Cancer could be thought of as a group of cells performing too well.

The built-in control mechanism that tells a cell to stop multiplying has somehow gotten its signals crossed. The result is run-away cell growth that can eventually have severe consequences. And yet, overproduction seems to be found everywhere in development, followed by "a pruning back of the branches of surviving cells," as William Calvin, neurobiologist and professor at the University of Washington, author of *In Search Of The Brain's Voice*, explains: *"All you need for cancer is failure to prune.* What's interesting about this is the unusual growth and control that's going on all over your body all the time. Perhaps there's really no such thing as perfect health, just periods of time when all this microscopic backing and filling is hidden from view."[1]

As long as intercellular signalling and immune systems are functioning well, cancer continues to be under control in a healthy human body. Many substances promote or accelerate cell growth, and many more help to control it. Estrogen is one that encourages growth. It has been referred to as "the hormone for beginnings," or, "the hormone of life." This conveys an idea of the power of estrogen but also its danger in the context of cancer.

There is no question that excessive estrogen may increase the risk of endometrial cancer (cancer of the lining of the uterus).[2] In 1984, the National Institute of Health Consensus Development Conference on Osteoporosis issued an official statement concerning endometrial cancer and ERT.

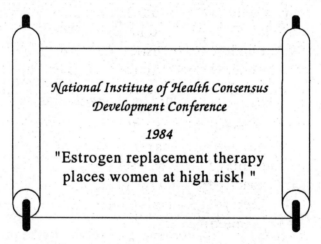

National Institute of Health Consensus Development Conference

1984

"Estrogen replacement therapy places women at high risk! "

The conference acknowledged the high risk of estrogen replacement therapy, but made an outrageous (in my opinion) statement about its possible side effect: "Estrogen-associated endometrial cancer is usually manifested at an early stage and is rarely fatal when managed appropriately."[3]

Great. It's okay if you get cancer—then the good doctor can zap you with radiation and chemotherapy to keep you from dying.

Research varies as to whether or not estradiol and estrone (forms of estrogen) are tumorogenic and carcinogenic.[4] Controversy no doubt stems from lack of consideration of excesses and/or synthetic forms of estrogens in many of the studies. Orally-administered estradiol is converted to estrone before being absorbed during digestion. *We must understand that estrogens don't initiate cancer; they can, however, promote it.*

Remember DES, a synthetic estrogen administered between 1945 and 1971 to help prevent miscarriages? There's a tragically high risk of vaginal cancer in girls whose mothers had DES treatment. (Turns out it was a useless and needless drug anyway.) In addition to cancer risk for females, males whose mothers were exposed to DES developed with undescended testicles. DES-exposed males may be less masculine because the undescended testicle interrupts the production of testosterone. Newest findings (*Lancet*, May 1993) report that males also have decreased semen volume and sperm counts. And there is even some evidence that exposed females may be masculinized.[5] You can see that when prenatal hormone environments are atypical, powerful influences come into play.[6] Do you really want to artificially promote the "capacity for growth" in *all* your tissues? Only if you can also keep your control systems functioning at full potential at the same time.

Because women can become pregnant during the few years prior to menopause, the possibility of starting any kind of synthetic hormonal therapy too early must be considered with care.

Although there is little doubt that estrogens are potent mammary tumor promoters when present in surplus amounts, the action of such transformation is poorly understood.[7] Studies support the notion that female hormones—when superfluous and synthetic—play a role in the development of brain tumors.[8]

FOOD SOURCES OF HORMONES

A mounting body of evidence suggests that other sources of estrogen contribute to the background level of carcinogens in our food environment. Milk, commercial eggs, and other dairy products often have traces of estrogen. Most commercial-grade meat is laced with it. Birth control pills are based on it—all piled on top of the other carcinogens accumulating in our environment.

Veterinary drugs have been regarded as necessary when producing food of animal origin. Keep in mind, however, that drug residues may persist in such foods and that there are problems associated with the use of hormonal or hormone-related compounds endowed with growth-promoting properties.

> According to a published 1991 review of drug practices in animals, *the current use of hormone compounds for "improved" food production does not rest on solid scientific ground.*[9]

Are you aware that when you buy a bottle of milk it usually comes from a cow that has been given growth hormone to enhance its milk yield?[10] In addition, hormones from the hypothalamus, pituitary, thyroid, adrenals, pancreas, and gonads, as well as related substances such as prostaglandins and growth factors, have been detected in milk. Exposure to prolactin in milk consumed by a pregnant woman occasionally shows deleterious long-term effects on mammary glands of offspring. Milk prolactin may also retard the preweaning growth, hasten puberty, control certain neuronal activity and influence the fluid absorption of offspring.[11]

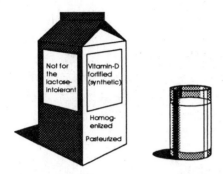

Many foods promoted as healthful are highly processed and may not be in your best health interest.

Foods which are healthful for some people can be very harmful for others.

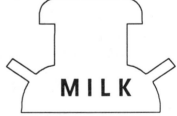

MILK

This product may be hazardous to your health!

Did you know that substances are used to manipulate the fatty acid profiles in cows? The goal is to produce lean meat! Biologically active residues all too frequently result from illegal treatment of animals sold for food in the market-place![12] You are protected to a small extent by the FDA and your liver. What? The FDA and your liver? Yes, but neither has what it takes for total command—that is, sufficient police power for the FDA to examine *all* markets, or the nutrients necessary for *first-pass removal* by your liver.

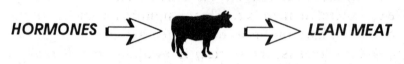

HORMONES ⇒ 🐄 ⇒ **LEAN MEAT**

Commentary on the possible effect of hormones in food on human growth was reported in *Medical Hypotheses*, 1992. According to studies noted by Dr. N. Moishezon-Blank, the practice of adding hormones to food may render one's liver incapable of efficient first-pass removal.

Changes in the shape and size of young Americans' heads show a tendency toward a decrease in size!

Moishezon-Blank and colleagues also suggest that the general acceleration of growth in the most recent American generation could be caused by accumulated hormone residues in the diet. Affecting long bones more than any other tissue, these residues also trigger inhibitors of growth during earlier stages of flat bone development. Consequently, the relative size of the skull (a flat bone structure), with respect to the body, is diminished. A reduction in the absolute size of the skull as well may accompany the change of body/head proportion.[13] Wouldn't you like to see more studies to validate these observations?

Hormone residues in milk may contribute to the increased height of the new generation of Asian Americans.

It should be noted that *estriol* is a form of estrogen that does not appear to be carcinogenic. This hormone may even have protective effects.[14] A healthy liver should convert estrone and estradiol to estriol, but the conversion may not always be complete. So there's risk that a significant amount of the potentially harmful forms of estrogen will get through. The safe form (that is, the estriol) is available for therapy in Europe, but not in North America.

Although today's medical journals frequently advocate hormone replacement therapy for each and every woman, occasionally a more balanced view appears. The *International Journal Of Fertility* proclaimed the following in 1989:

> *Not all postmenopausal women need estrogen replacement. Some continue to produce significant amounts of their own estrogens, many need progestogen replacement to reduce the risk for endometrial hyperplasia [abnormal increase of cells associated with cancer] and cancer itself. Where estrogen therapy retards the development of and helps to prevent osteoporosis, added progestogen may restore bone which has been lost by promoting new bone formation.*[15]

When you read or are told about safety features of "new" hormone therapies, remember that they are usually compared with their more harmful counterparts currently or formerly in use, rather than with natural modalities.

MORE ABOUT ERT AND SIDE EFFECTS

Here's a summary of possible (if not usual) side effects of ERT:

> Abdominal cramps
> Amenorrhea
> Bloating
> Breast tenderness and enlargement
> Cystitis-like syndromes
> Elevated blood pressure
> Endometrial cancer
> Gallbladder disease
> Hair loss
> Hyperlipidemia
> Jaundice
> Mental depression
> Nausea and vomiting
> Prolonged vaginal bleeding
> Reduced carbohydrate tolerance
> Reduced glucose tolerance
> Skin rashes
> Thrombophlebitis
> Undesirable weight gain or loss
> Vaginal candidiasis[16,17,18]

Reflect on this list. Then note this quotation from the pages of *Senior Patient*, a subsidiary of *Postgraduate Medicine*:

> *It now seems reasonable to recommend that all postmenopausal women—regardless of age or symptoms—be seriously considered for hormone replacement therapy. The disadvantages are not necessarily medically risky, but are a matter of patients' attitudes.*[19]

Huh? A matter of *attitude*? Here we go again!

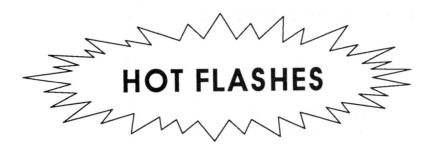

HOT FLASHES

➤ A Western diet elevates levels of sex hormones, increasing harmful steroids.
> *Scandinavian Journal of Clinical and Laboratory Investigation*, 1990[20]

➤ Estrogen replacement increases the risk of endometrial cancer during treatment and for many years after it is discontinued.
> *Obstetrics and Gynecology*, 1990[21]

➤ Evidence supporting estrogen's role in breast cancer comes from international studies.
> *Breast Cancer Research and Treatment*, 1991[22]

➤ A Western diet increases levels of sex hormones, resulting in decreased formation of mammalian compounds which could protect against cancer-cell growth.
> *Scandinavian Journal of Clinical and Laboratory Investigation*, 1990[23]

➤ The risk of breast cancer could be reduced by minimizing the therapeutic use of estrogens and progestogens in postmenopausal women.
> *Journal of Cancer and Clinical Oncology*, 1988[24]

➤ Cervical cancer is stimulated in response to excess estradiol.
> *International Journal of Cancer*, 1992[25]

➤ Estradiol-17 beta is associated with breast cancer.

Breast Cancer Research and Treatment, 1992[26]

➤ Lab studies suggest that some androgenic hormones stimulate cancer in bladder tissue.

Cancer Causes and Control, 1992[27]

➤ Estrogen influences the development of gall-bladder cancer.

Medical Hypotheses, 1991[28]

➤ Sex hormones may have a role in broncho-genic carcinoma.

Cancer Research, 1990[29]

➤ The potential for pancreatic cancer can be demonstrated after hormonal manipulations.

International Journal of Pancreatology, 1990[30]

➤ Significant stimulation of certain gastric and colorectal cells occur with large concentrations of estradiol.

Cancer, 1989[31]

➤ Estrogen therapy may contribute to breast cancer because the mammary gland is already oversaturated with estrogens.

Revue Francaise de Gynecologie et D Obstetrique, 1991[32]

➤ There is direct evidence of a relationship between lowered spatial ability and prenatal exposure to DES in males.

Hormones and Behavior, 1992[33]

~~ ENDNOTES ~~ *The fantasy continues...*

We affirm that hormone therapy could, for a time, slow the process of bone loss. We affirm that there are certain risks involved.

Our fantasy reveals an exciting surprise! We didn't think we could rebuild bone once osteoporosis left its calling card, did we? But look at those osteoblasts—they're gobbling up the progesterone and *empowering new bone construction, enough to make up for long-time deprivation!* It's a slow process, rather like watching grass grow.

If we put our fantasy on fast forward, we can see it happen —*not to those without the progesterone, however.* See how much more efficiently bone growth comes about when we add special nutrients.

And look! It's even happening to that much older woman. Wow!

~~~

One of the first symptoms of osteoporosis is often loss of height. The progressive decrease in bone mass results in this gradual loss and

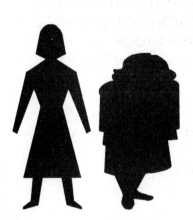

eventual "dow-a g e r's hump." This is known as *kyphosis.* The hunch-back look is caused by the abnormally in-creased convex shape in the spine's curvature.

It doesn't have to be this way!

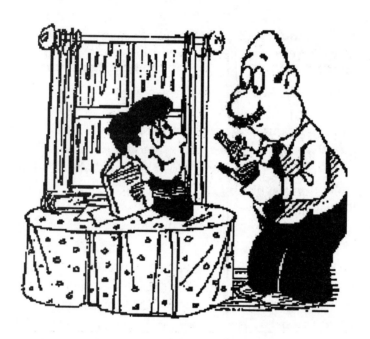

Hurry up and bring me a glass of milk
before my doctor changes his mind about it.

9

NATURAL PROGESTERONE

The dangers of estrogen replacement therapy are only part of the problem. *Early researchers in this area were not looking at all the facts.* No one paid much attention to the research showing that progesterone tapers off at about the same time that the process of osteoporosis begins, *followed* by the decline of estrogen.

> There seems to be no good reason to have chosen estrogen over progesterone as the hormone of replacement.

In fact, the sequence of the decline of progesterone, beginning several years before menopause when estrogen sufficiency persists, correlates even better than estrogen with the onset of osteoporosis.

That statement was made by John R. Lee, M.D. Dr. Lee is a practitioner in Northern California who has had significant success reversing osteoporosis in his patients![1]

But we still strive for facts which are more than guilt by association. We need to understand just what estrogen and progesterone are doing to your bones, and some awareness may finally be surfacing. Jerilynn Prior, M.D., of the Endocrinology and Metabolism Division of the University of British Columbia, is believed to have identified the roles of these hormones in bone remodelling. Estrogen may reduce the rate of bone loss by reducing the activity of *osteoclasts*, the cells that *resorb* calcium phosphate back into your blood plasma. (Resorption refers to calcium leaving your bone and re-entering your blood.) Progesterone, on the other hand, actually works in conjunction with *osteoblasts*, the cells associated with building new bone material.

Typical of so many revelations, Dr. Prior's awareness of progesterone's role in bone health came about accidentally. She was measuring the estrogen and progesterone levels of female athletes. The results were unrelated to her expectations; she discovered that the athletes who had low progesterone but high estrogen levels showed signs of osteoporosis. How could this be? Wasn't it an established fact that estrogen *deficiency* causes osteoporosis? Could this mean that *progesterone* deficiency is the culprit?

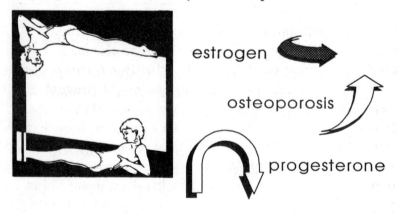

estrogen

osteoporosis

progesterone

Dr. Prior's suspicions were confirmed. She explains:

> *Progesterone binds to receptors on osteo-blasts, increases the rate of bone formation and remodelling when given therapeutically to oophorectomized dogs [dogs whose ovaries are removed], and slows bone loss in postmenopausal women. Progesterone acts on bone, even though estrogen activity is low or absent. Because progesterone appears to work on the osteoblast to increase bone formation, it would complement the actions of estrogen to decrease bone resorption.[2]*

In other words, progesterone builds bone!

Dr. Prior cites additional validation in a letter published in the *New England Journal of Medicine*, 1993:

> *Evidence that progesterone acts as a bone-trophic [stimulating] hormone has recently been extended by work documenting the presence of progesterone receptors on osteo-blasts.[3]*

Studies on both animals and humans show that progestogens have a growth-promoting effect on bone tissue. Research with nonmenopausal women treated with *natural progesterone* suggests that such a hormone might prevent bone loss![4] This explains why ERT alone yields limited results. Estrogen can reduce the rate of bone loss, but bone loss is only one problem. In view of the risks, doesn't it make more sense to work on supplying more *new bone material* instead of just reducing the rate of bone loss? (It's one thing to spend less money and slow the decline of your bank account. It's quite another to replace the money spent to keep the balance stable.)

Dr. Lee validates these results clinically. He recounts success in actually *reversing* osteoporosis, instead of merely arresting its progress. This excerpt is from his paper published in *Medical Hypothesis* in 1991, summarizing results of his treatment plan:

> *Since 1982, I have followed 100 patients, all post-menopausal white women (average age 65.2 years, range 38 to 83 years) in a suburban setting. The average time from menopause was 16 years. The majority had already noted height loss, a cardinal sign of osteoporosis, and many had experienced one or more fractures. The benefits from the treatment program were so obvious to these patients that no problems with patient compliance arose. Nor were any side effects or adverse alterations in blood lipids observed. Each patient was followed a minimum of three years.*
>
> *In the study group of 100 patients, height loss was stabilized, previous musculoskeletal aches and pains disappeared and no osteoporotic fractures occurred. Three traumatic fractures did occur and, in each case, these healed normally with the treating orthopedist commenting on the good quality of their bones.*
>
> *In the major sub-group of 63 patients with...bone density tests, the average three-year change in density actually increased 15.4 percent, instead of losing an expected 4.5 percent.*[5]

One must be impressed with Dr. Lee's human trials and their very encouraging outcomes. They strongly suggest that osteoporosis can be reversed. Significantly, Dr. Lee found that age does not seem to be a determinant—70-year-old patients experience the same increase in bone density as younger women. As is usually the case with adaptogenic natural treatments (rather than symptom-suppressing therapies), those with the lowest bone densities experience the *greatest* relative improvement. (See Table 2 below.)

TABLE 2
DR. LEE'S DATA:
BONE DENSITY IMPROVEMENT
WITH PROGESTERONE

Lumbar Bone Mass Density (gm/sq cm)	Initial Average	3-Year Average	% Gain
0.5-0.8	0.745	0.911	22.8
0.8-0.9	0.838	0.992	18.4
0.9-1.0	0.957	1.122	17.2
1.0-1.1	1.026	1.134	10.5
1.1-1.2	1.152	1.215	5.5
1.2-1.3	1.256	1.289	2.6

What did Dr. Lee do to achieve his remarkable success? Diet, vitamins, exercise, and a combination of estrogen and natural progesterone were all part of his bone-loss-prevention blue-print. The dietary changes, interestingly, emphasized green leafy vegetables as a calcium source rather than the traditional dairy products. This makes sense in view of the high incidence of lactose intolerance (inability to digest milk sugars), a problem that intensifies as we get older. (Blacks and Asians face this problem in their teens; northern

Europeans at the adult level.) Red meat was limited to three times per week, sodas avoided, cigarettes not allowed at all, and alcohol severely curbed.

The daily vitamin and food supplements included:

> ➤ 350-400 I.U. vitamin D
> ➤ 2,000 milligrams vitamin C divided into several doses throughout the day
> ➤ 25,000 I.U. beta-carotene (a form of vitamin A)
> ➤ 800-1,000 milligrams calcium

None of these doses is particularly high.

0.3 to 0.625 milligrams per day of conjugated estrogen was taken for three weeks each month. (Conjugated estrogen is a mixture of estrogenic substances that are of the type excreted by pregnant mares, as in Premarin, prepared to enhance absorption.)

Natural progesterone, in a three-percent cream, was applied to the skin under the arms, neck, breasts, belly, and face (alternately) before bed twelve days during the last two weeks of monthly estrogen use.

Except for the estrogen and progesterone, the above regimen is perfectly sensible for virtually anybody who wants to improve overall health. The vitamin doses are moderate.

The dietary recommendations suggested by Dr. Lee correspond to what I've been trying to get my family and friends to do for most of my life!

But are the hormones really necessary? That depends. Dr. Lee acknowledges the absence of a control group and a double-blind study at this early stage. He points out, however, that the conventional treatment programs—those that use estrogen alone—constitute a kind of *real-world* control group, and the results obtained are not nearly as positive. In fact, a recent report in *Lancet*, 1993, shows that long-term estrogen therapy is difficult for both doctors and their patients to accept, as has been confirmed by the very high degree of noncompliance.[6]

> Unlike estrogen therapy, the application of natural progesterone in a cream base has met with success.

Dr. Lee cites three studies indicating that synthetic progestogen treatment by itself may have a bone-restoring effect, but the results present complications.

(1) Double-blind, placebo-controlled research involving 84 postmenopausal women over a two-year time period was conducted. It was found that while the overall bone loss was no greater for a progestogen-only group, certain specific bone tissues seemed to lose less material with the use of estrogen only.[7,8]

(2) Another similar study by the same researchers demonstrated synthetic progestogen alone to be equivalent to estrogen alone.

(3) And in Dr. Prior's own clinical observations involving postmenopausal women with endocrine disorders that precluded estrogen treatment, the patients all experienced an increase in vertebral bone density after one year on medroxyprogesterone, 10 milligrams per day.[9]

Medroxyprogesterone is the most widely used synthetic progesterone, as in Provera.

Test results of these studies may have been different and more dramatic if not for one factor: *the research included the use of oral, synthetic progestogens.* Recall that progesterone is subject to destruction on the first pass through your liver. Some researchers claim that the natural *transdermal* form of application (application and absorption on and through your skin, usually as a cream), is the best way to bypass this possible roadblock. Recall Dr. Lee's success. Others insist that oral forms can be extremely potent. Both forms are easily available in the United States. (Check with your physician or your local health store.)

In his book, *Nutrition for Women,* biologist Raymond Peat, Ph.D., of Eugene, Oregon, advocates the transdermal method of administering progesterone as superior to oral, injection, suppository, or sublingual methods.[10]

An interesting study by Joel Hargrove, M.D., of the Obstetrics and Gynecology Department of Vanderbuilt University Medical Center, compares the use of natural progesterone and estradiol with that of synthetic progesterone (medroxyprogesterone acetate) and conjugated estrogens.[11] Four perimenopausal women and thirteen postmenopausal women sought treatment for symptoms related to menopause. They volunteered for the 12-month study. Results are shown in Table 3 on page 117.

TABLE 3
COMPARISON OF TWO THERAPIES:
Estradiol with Progesterone
and
Conjugated Estrogens with Medroxyprogesterone

Symptoms	estradiol and natural progesterone		conjugated estrogens and medroxyprogesterone	
	Baseline (before treatment)	12 months later	Baseline (before treatment)	12 months later
Hot flashes	9	0	5	3
Night sweats	6	0	4	3
Insomnia	4	1	3	1
Decreased libido	6	0	2	0
Vaginal dryness	5	0	3	2
Anxiety	6	3	3	1
Depression	1	1	3	0

Here's another impressive success rate. Look at the difference between the two treatments. The combination of pure (or natural progesterone) and estradiol is noticeably more effective than the more traditional mix of conjugated estrogen and medroxyprogesterone acetate.

So it's not always enough to talk about estrogen and progesterone. One must be very specific about the *form* in which these substances are administered. Of course, the study makes no attempt to determine which of the two variables in each part of the test was the more important one—the natural progesterone or the estradiol; the synthetic progestogen or the conjugated estrogen. I have my suspicions, but we await additional hard data from clinical trials.

Despite the possible advantages of adding progestogens to estrogen therapy (inforamtion cited consistently across medical publications today), 40 to 60 percent of physicians in this country are still prescribing unopposed estrogen![12] (Unopposed estrogen refers to the use of estrogen without the balance of progesterone, synthetic *or* natural.) Furthermore, the physicians who even *think* of checking for progesterone levels are few and far between.

Martin Milner, N.D., a naturopathic physician in Portland, Oregon, reports that not a single patient complaining of PMS or menopausal symptoms ever had a progesterone level determined by any of the physicians she had consulted before coming to his office.[13] (Dr. Milner has been in practice 11 years.)

As stated in *Endocrine Reviews*, 1990, past researchers appeared to be prophetic when they commented:

Osteoporosis may be, in part, a progesterone-deficiency disease.[14]

¤

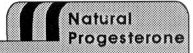

MEMOS

Facts and Functions of Natural Progesterone

Progesterone is a female sex hormone, also found in males.

Natural progesterone:
➤ is also manufactured by the testes in males and adrenal cortex in males and females
➤ helps to regulate accessory organs during the menstrual cycle
➤ prepares the uterus for the implantation of the blastocyst (the embryo)
➤ has LDL cholesterol as its precursor in luteal tissue
➤ is secreted by the corpus luteum following the discharge of the ovum (if no fertilization takes place)
➤ may reach a production rate during the luteal phase of 30 milligrams a day
➤ falls abruptly 10 to 12 days after ovulation, followed by the onset of menstruation
➤ helps to maintain pregnancy
➤ rises to 300 milligrams a day (by placenta) during the third trimester

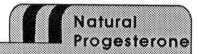

MEMOS

Natural Progesterone

Natural progesterone (continued):

➤ is carried in the blood by binding with cortisol-binding globulin
➤ can be measured to confirm ovulation
➤ levels in saliva can determine its luteal function
➤ has specific functions not found in any other compound
➤ can be produced synthetically and is then called progestin, gestagen, or a progestational agent
➤ shares only the ability to sustain human secretory endometrium with synthetic progestogens (no synthetic progesterone has the full spectrum of natural progesterone's biologic activity)
➤ is used for birth control pills and hormone replacement therapy in the synthetic form
➤ reduces the fibrocystic breast condition, which occurs because of continued estrogen dominance
➤ regulates salt retention (but does not increase sodium and water content, as do most progestins)
➤ modulates nerve function

MEMOS

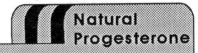

Natural progesterone (continued)

➤ promotes healthy thymus glands
➤ is suppressed by continuous progestins
➤ has a far greater positive effect on bone building in postmenopausal women than progestins, even though some progestins do have some bone-building benefit
➤ functions as a mild antidepressant
➤ is safe, unlike synthetic progestins, all of which have a wide variety of side effects
➤ can be as beneficial when applied transdermally as by oral administration

Progesterone, usually in a synthetic form, has been prescribed for:
* amenorrhea
* dysmenorrhea
* endometriosis
* funtional uterine bleeding
* premenstrual tension
* threatened or habitual abortion

The following synthetic progestins are in use:
Delalutin — hydroxyprogesterone caproate in oil
Provera — methoxyprogesterone acetate
Norlutin — norethindrone

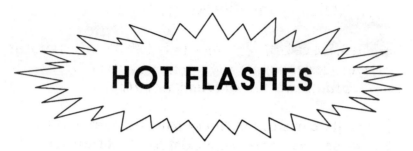

HOT FLASHES

➢ Progesterone alone may be a valuable agent for management of postmenopausal osteoporosis.

Journal of Bone and Mineral Research, 1990[15]

➢ Progesterone may influence skeletal metabolism.

American Journal of Obstetrics and Gynecology, 1992[16]

➢ Progesterone promotes bone formation and/or increases bone turnover.

Endocrine Reviews, 1990[17]

➢ Progesterone meets the necessary criteria to play a causal role in mineral metabolism.

Endocrine Reviews, 1990[18]

➢ The addition of a progestogen helps to protect against long-term effects of unopposed estrogen on the endometrium.

American Journal of Obstetrics and Gynecology, 1992[19]

➢ Postmenopausal women with benign and malignant ovarian tumors have low progesterone levels prior to surgery.

Acta Endocrinologica, 1992[20]

~~ ENDNOTES ~~ *The fantasy continues...*

Intrigued, we can see that when fatty fish, eggs, butter, and liver are ingested, calcium absorption is more efficient. *Not so with sodas, unleavened bread, or milk.*

Cow's milk contains four times more calcium than human milk, and so we watch, perplexed, as the breast-fed baby absorbs more calcium than the child who is fed cow's milk! We are amazed when the oxalic acid in spinach, Swiss chard, beet greens, and parsley casts a spell over calcium, rendering it less absorbable.

If the experts cannot sort it out, how can we?

Hormone replacement therapy is not the only area of serious controversy when it comes to the accepted methods of dealing with osteoporosis. Misinformation surrounding calcium absorption and supplementation runs a close second.

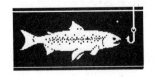

Helps calcium absorption!

Hinders calcium absorption!

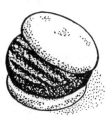

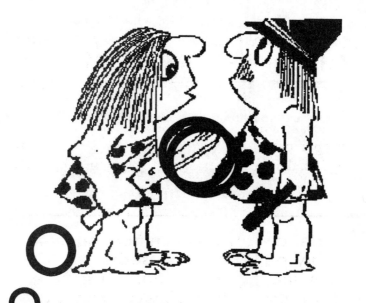

I just invented the wheel.
But I know that a few centuries
from now, you men will take all
the credit.

10

WHAT ABOUT CALCIUM SUPPLEMENTS?

If calcium loss is a major part of the problem and we can't get the proper calcium absorption from our modern-day diets, does it make sense to eat more calcium in supplemental form?

> Consider dietary calcium from an evolutionary perspective—researchers tell us that the prevailing calcium intake during most of human evolution was substantially higher than it is today.[1] (No surprises here.)

So taking supplemental calcium in the form of tablets or capsules appears to be an obvious course of action to help guard against osteoporosis. But for reasons that are still not entirely clear, calcium supplementation for the purpose of improving bone integrity has been largely ineffective. Let's explore what we do know in this area.

An editorial in *New England Journal of Medicine*, 1993, summarizes the situation:

> *For the past ten years, both scientists and the lay public have been subjected to a spate of claims and counterclaims about the value of ensuring an adequate intake of calcium throughout life. Although the role of calcium supplements in the health of adult bone has been called controversial, it may be more accurate to say that it has been confusing. A recent review identified 43 studies published since 1988 that relate calcium intake to bone mass, bone loss, or bone fragility. Twenty-six reported that calcium intake is associated in some way with bone mass, bone loss, or fracture; 16 do not. In a presidential election, such a majority would be considered a landslide, but for scientists, the 16 negative studies leave a nagging doubt. Does that difference mean that calcium is less important, or perhaps not important at all?[2]*

This very year, *Lancet* stated that there is no convincing evidence that a high calcium intake will substantially affect bone loss.[3] *New England Journal of Medicine* reports that no published study sheds useful light on the question of *how much* calcium is needed for bone health.[4] The *Southern Medical Journal* advises that increased calcium intake in supplemental form will *not* increase skeletal mass in mature, premenopausal women and will not prevent bone loss in postmenopausal women.[5] *Bone and Mineral* concludes that because iron, zinc and magnesium intake are positively correlated with forearm bone mass content in pre-menopausal women, *bone mass is influenced by dietary factors other than calcium.*[6]

Another important finding is that calcium *by itself* somehow interferes with vitamin D in its hormonal form. Henry DeLuca M.D., known for his research on vitamin D, writes in *Complimentary Medicine*:

> *The emphasis on calcium has taken the focus away from the complexity of the issue and is preventing some kinds of therapy. For example, treatment with the hormonal form of vitamin D cannot be administered with high intakes of calcium.*
>
> *We tear down our skeleton and build it back about once every five years. If you take large amounts of calcium, you turn off the production of the hormone. That interferes with bone remodeling.*
>
> *I believe it is okay to take extra calcium, but I don't think anyone should be misled into believing that if she or he has osteoporosis, taking calcium is going to help or cure.*[7]

Two warnings come to mind:

(1) If you have seen references to (or your physician tells you about) a study reported in *New England Journal of Medicine* extolling the benefits of 1500 milligrams of supplemental calcium per day, take heed. A careful researcher will note that the study reveals that it took at least two years for any significant results to surface; that the percentage of increased bone density was within the range of error of the testing machines; and that the women were still losing bone. *The loss was simply less than losses compared with other women.* Again, we need to be aware of the parameters used as guidelines.

(2) Don't throw the baby out with the bath water. Calcium supplementation has other advantages. Significant bone preservation during menopausal years just doesn't appear to be one of them—unless you are truly calcium deficient. Note, too, that many studies are not done with a sharp enough pencil. *It may be that certain forms of calcium, combined with other specific nutrients, produce different results.* For example, it has been reported in *Calcification Tissue International*, 1992, that supplemental calcium with vitamin D appears to reduce hip and other nonvertebral fractures in the elderly.[8] And hydrochloric acid can be as necessary as vitamin D for healthy bones. For efficient absorption, calcium supplementation MUST be taken with synergistic nutrients, discussed in a later chapter.

FIGURE 15

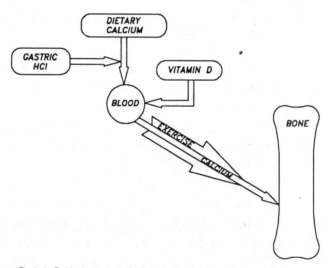

CALCIUM ABSORPTION HELPERS

Gastric hydrochloric acid (HCl) helps the absorption of dietary calcium. Vitamin D is necessary to incorporate calcium into bone structure. And the bone-building process is greatly accelerated by exercise.

Even injecting calcium directly into the bloodstream has little effect on bone health.[9]

The amount of available calcium, dietary or in blood, is not the limiting factor in your ability to maintain the integrity of your bones. (See Figure 15 on page 128.)

When areas of the world with notably low dietary calcium (the South African Bantu region, Hong Kong, and Singapore) are compared with high calcium populations (Britain, Sweden, and the United States), it becomes obvious that high calcium intake alone is not associated with long-lasting healthy bones.[10]

The *Journal of Internal Medicine*, 1992, reports that although quite a number of calcium supplements are available, many are marketed without proper knowledge of the bioavailability of the actual preparation.[11] This could provide different results and lead to controversy among the researchers.

Clearly, there are factors at work other than calcium, and there is still a lot to be learned. But much information is already available. Those of us who have examined the research and clinical results have at least an inkling of what does make a difference. The good news is that many of these factors are easily within your control.

¤

MEMOS

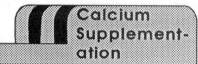
Calcium Supplement- ation

NOTES ON CALCIUM SUPPLEMENTATION

Despite the controversy concerning calcium supplementation, most practitioners advise its use. They understand that absorption varies considerably, since calcium absorption is dependent on vitamin D intake, exercise, and a host of additional factors, known and unknown. Until more is understood, practitioners deem it appropriate to attempt to insure nutritional status by recommending intakes of 800 to 1,200 milligrams daily. One gets the impression that it is being prescribed as a safeguard, "just in case." (You're not superstitious, but you don't walk under a ladder.)

If you decide to continue calcium supplementation and increase the dosage to 1,200 or 1,500 milligrams, magnesium supplementation should be increased in equal amounts. Single tablets containing equal amounts of both substances are available. Magnesium improves calcium retention. Calcium also reduces zinc. If you take calcium and zinc supplements separately, you may enhance retention of each.

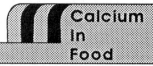

MEMOS

Calcium
In
Food

NOTES ON CALCIUM IN FOODS

Two large dried figs contain 80 milli-grams of calcium, but it takes 156 sal-tine crackers to render the same 80 milligrams. One portion of raw green vegetables can have up to 250 milli-grams of calcium. (Summer vegetables, by the way, have more calcium than fall or winter vegetables.) Four ounces of salmon contain 291 milligrams of cal-cium, but it takes 485 saltines, or 73 cups of cornflakes (without milk) to fill you with the same 291 milligrams.

Foods that decrease calcium absorp-tion are cocoa, bran, and wheat germ.

Butterfat promotes the absorption of calcium. The fat content of one or two or even three glasses of whole milk daily, as compared with skimmed or low-fat milk, will not affect your weight or your cholesterol levels, as advertisements have suggested. (The major culprit is *processed* dairy fat.)

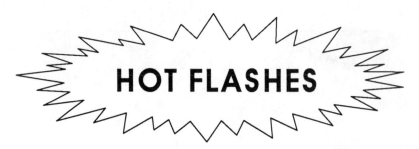

HOT FLASHES

➤ Recommendations for bone integrity, such as calcium supplementation, are of little value and are inconsistent with available studies.
   Medical Hypotheses, 1988[12]

➤ Substantial bone loss occurs in women despite intake of 750 milligrams of calcium daily.
   New England Journal of Medicine, 1993[13]

➤ Little evidence supports the effectiveness of calcium as a strategy to prevent hip fractures.
   Lancet, 1993[14]

➤ The role of calcium intake in preventing osteoporosis remains a matter of debate.
   Wiener Medizinische Wochenschrift, 1990[15]

➤ Large intakes of dietary calcium can cause constipation.
   Annual Review of Nutrition, 1990[16]

➤Japanese, with lower bone density and lower calcium intake, experience far less fractures than we do.
   Proceedings of the Society for Experimental Biology and Medicine, 1992[17]

Other studies demonstrating similar results have been published in *New England Journal of Medicine, Lancet,* and *American Journal of Medicine.*[18,19,20,21]

~~ ENDNOTES ~~ *The fantasy continues...*

My fantasy transports us to Brazil's southeastern Atlantic forest, where we study the menu of a monkey—the *muriquis*. This primate self-medicates. The purpose of our junket is to see *how* and try to discern *why*.

We note that from late September to mid-October, when banquets of edible fruit abound, the muriquis monkeys eat mainly the leaves of only two plants of the legume family. The monkeys actually camp out at the leaf sources, behaving as if these leaves were the most delectable of all fruits. (They are not.) And then they seek another fruit, known as *monkey ear*. But here they take only small nibbles, as we might do when sampling a strange hors d'oeuvre at a cocktail party.

Ordinarily, the muriquis prefer more succulent fruits, even if it takes a greater effort to locate them. So why the change in preference at this time of year? By eating the leguminous leaves instead of the fruits, both male and female appear to get a surge of protein, *which fortifies them for the upcoming mating season.*

But why the monkey ear fruit? Guess what! Monkey ear contains *stigmasterol*, a steroid used in the laboratory manufacture of progesterone! Recent studies indicate that plant hormones can regulate reproduction in some animals. It is suggested that stigmasterol is linked to the monkeys' seasonal fertility.[22]

Since we can dream anything, let's assume we have viewed the cellular structure of the foods consumed by the muriqui. Then let us bring this information to our own bodies to have more insight into what it is that we should be eating—and how *we, too,* can safely self-medicate.

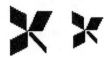 *Grandma's Recipe for Bone Soup*

Veal joints (knuckles) or young chicken bones, or beef neck, or any young cancellous (latticelike) bones

1 cup barley
2 to 3 quarts water
green vegetables in season
   (the more the better)
seasonings to taste

Cook bones and barley in water. Bring to boil and simmer over low heat ½ hour.

Nutrition Tip: No better soup for your aching bones!

11

FOOD AS SELF-MEDICATION

FEMALE AND FEELING FINE

There are easy measures you can take to keep your bones healthy and your hormones flowing properly. Best of all, these practices help to prevent discomfort. You should also understand that although discomfort is typical, it is definitely not normal.

Some of these steps are easy, although some may tax your powers of self-discipline to the limit. No two individuals respond exactly the same way, and any of these suggestions could turn out to be critical for you. And keep in mind that unlike drugs, natural procedures for turning things around don't work instantly. You didn't lose bone density in a day. So give nature a little time here. Young or old, you *can* turn things around!

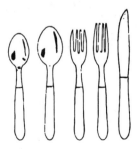 What you put in your mouth every day of your life, affects the length and quality of your entire life.

Eat Your Vegetables

Eat your veggies! Simple advice, and timeless. Green leafy vegetables are your best source of calcium. Far better than milk, as it turns out.

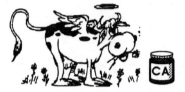

Where does all that calcium in milk come from, anyway? Do you see the farmer giving calcium pills to the cows?

This is a key element of Dr. Lee's regimen, with which he has had outstanding success for reversing osteoporosis. Perhaps veggies work as a good source of calcium because of the co-factor nutrients they contain, such as silicon, boron, beta-carotene, and even vitamin C. These nutrients are discussed in detail in the next segment. Vegetables may work more efficiently because they are a more direct source of calcium; the cow eats the stuff that grows in the ground, makes the milk, and you drink the milk. Why not eat the food that grows in the ground to begin with? Maybe it's like taping a video from another video, rather than buying the original. Each copy "loses a generation," reducing quality. An oversimplification, but you get the point.

Avoid Dairy Products

Avoiding dairy products may fly in the face of conventional wisdom. Cow's milk is a perfect food—*for a calf!* Humans were never designed to drink cow's milk. In this country, with such an abundance of healthful food choices available, milk should be considered as a slightly more subtle kind of junk food, to be avoided or used in very limited quantities. Low-fat and non-fat milk, surprisingly, are even worse.

> The fat in milk plays an important part in the digestion and assimilation of other nutrients in milk—*including calcium!* Drinking low-fat or no-fat milk is not in your best health interest.

A very high percentage of North Americans are lactose-intolerant to some degree and should avoid milk for other health reasons. Half the diabetics in this country are milk sensitive. Casein (the protein portion of milk) binds minerals. *Because of its high level of animal protein, milk consumption may cause greater calcium loss than gain.*[1]

Interestingly, homogenization makes the situation much worse. Particles of milk fat are drastically reduced in size and increased in number as a result of homogenization, resulting in far more surface area to be acted on. The faster absorption rate of these tiny fat particles can be a problem. Unhomogenized milk is hard to find, but it is superior (or, more accurately, less damaging).

Fermented products with viable culture, such as the yogurt produced by nutrition-aware companies (available in health stores and an occasional supermarket), may be a more acceptable alternative. Try plain yogurt as a milk substitute on breakfast cereal, for example. Or substitute watered-down yogurt in recipes when milk is called for. Lactase (the lactose- or milk-metabolizing enzyme) is produced in the fermentation process, so fermented milk products are often tolerated by the milk-sensitive even though these foods are milk-based.

As stated earlier, there's also the danger that milk may add dietary estrogen and other hormones—now used freely in animals by the dairy industry. True, first-pass liver treatment attempts to remove these foreign hormones, but, as discussed, there is uncertainty as to how much of the unwanted constituents are ignored by your liver.

Avoid Junk Foods

You already know that you should avoid junk foods. Easier said than done, isn't it? Like many Americans, you may feel guilty when you consume them, but not guilty enough to abstain.

Does it surprise you that sugar affects your bones? If you are concerned about osteoporosis, perhaps you will be a little more selective when making food choices if you know that sugar increases calcium excretion.

Forty-four percent of patients with osteoporosis require complete dentures before the age of sixty, compared with only 15 percent of non-osteoporotic patients.

The teeth of osteoporotics don't degrade along with the bones. Teeth are built differently, and do not lose calcium or accept it the way healthy bones do. But there are different connections. The same dietary factors (including sugar consumption) that destroy teeth also take their toll on the rest of your body.

Avoid Junk Drinks

What's a junk drink? Almost everything except pure spring water. We've already discussed milk, and although this may be hard to accept, I have to classify cow's milk as a junk drink.

Sodas

Sodas are devastating to bone health because of their phosphorus content. When physicians study results of bone photon tests, they can actually identify the 18- and 19-year-olds who drink the colas.

Coffee

Coffee is dangerous because of its effect on pH balance. Dr. Corsello explains:

> *A good natural defense against osteoporosis is to keep the acidity of your blood in proper balance. If <u>you</u> don't, <u>your body</u> will, by removing calcium from your bones to defend the pH balance in your blood."[2] An interesting point! Also note that smoking, alcohol, and coffee all raise blood acidity.*

Coffee is a tough one because aside from its mild addictive quality, it is firmly entrenched in daily routines, if not in our culture. My personal conclusion is that coffee, along with the use of soft drinks, contributes more osteoporosis than current thinking acknowledges. I'm not waiting for more research. These drinks are out of my diet permanently.

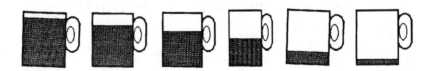

MEMOS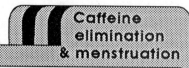

ABSTRACT: The rate at which caffeine is eliminated from the body decreases as the levels of sex steroids due to pregnancy or oral contraceptive use increase. [This may be why so many women can't drink coffee when pregnant.]

An investigation has now been made into whether the changes in sex steroid levels that occur during normal menstrual cycling also affect the rate of caffeine elimination. The evidence suggests that caffeine elimination may be slowed in the late luteal phase, prior to the onset of menstruation. Such a reduction leads to increased accumulation of caffeine with repeated self-administration during the day.

Lane JD; Steege JF; Rupp SL; Kuhn CM. Menstrual cycle effects on caffeine elimination in the human female. *European Journal of Clinical Pharmacology*, 1992, 43(5):543-6.

Fruit juice

Fruit drinks (even those to which sugar has NOT been added) are much too sweet—too high in simple carbohydrates—to be nutritionally valuable. Note the metabolic differences that occur when you consume apple juice, compared with eating whole apples containing the same number of calories:

After the apple juice:
- ➤ insulin responses are 50 percent greater
- ➤ you are hungry sooner
- ➤ your cholesterol levels are higher
- ➤ a rebound fall in glucose follows.

Ready-to-drink fruit juices may also have more fluoride than your body can handle comfortably. (See pages 142 and 156 for more information on fluoride.) The source, of course, is the water added to fruit concentrates.[3]

Hard to accept, isn't it, considering how long fruit juices have been promoted as healthful and "natural."
I'll confess that I still drink bottled fruit juice, but only in very small quantities. To make powdered and granulated supplements more palatable, I add about an inch of pure fruit juice to filtered water. I know, however, that when my blood chemistry begins to show the first signs of going askew, even that small amount of fruit juice will be deleted from my diet immediately.

So when it comes to fruit juice, moderation is good, but abstinence is best. Try to eat the whole fruit instead— it really is more satisfying. (If you must drink juices, avoid those that are packaged in aluminum cans. Glass containers are preferable.)

What About Other Liquids?

Fresh vegetable juices are another story. They can have tremendous therapeutic value, and if you're lucky enough to have a good juicer, there are times you want to put it to use.

Most vegetables contain good ratios of calcium and phosphorus, and some even have considerably more calcium than phosphorus. (The latter include alfalfa, parsley, dandelion greens, and chard, to name a few.)

Because the concentration of minerals in the American diet is not very high, you need to consume large quantities of vegetables to compensate for the offenses of your real-world diet. Juicing vegetables can help.

Cautions are necessary here, too, however. Vegetable juice degenerates nutritionally with incredible speed —it's been claimed that the "half-life" of a glass of carrot juice is only 12 minutes. Additional problems: carrot juice kept at room temperature for 24 hours has unfavorable concentrations of carcinogenic nitrites.[4]

And isn't juice itself unnatural? How can we justify drinking a liquid that contains 10 or 20 times the amount of nutrients than would be found in the unprocessed vegetables? And what about the fiber that gets lost in the juicing process? These are valid concerns, and that's why I eat most of my vegetables whole. Vegetable juices can be *therapeutic*; whole vegetables can be preventive.

So we're left with water. Oh, did I mention fluoridation? Fluoride therapy was once considered potentially beneficial for the treatment of osteoporosis because it increases bone mass. Fluoride, however, is deleterious to connective tissue, causing a wide assortment of ligament, tendon, periarticular (situated around a joint), and bone problems.[5]

"I'm getting thirsty.
What kind of bottled water
does your mother buy?"

Fluoride may increase *bone mass*, but it does nothing to increase bone *strength*. Think of an old concrete bridge, with the concrete now dry and brittle. You can make the roadway thicker by adding a layer of gravel to the surface. Surveys will show more mass and more material. But have you made the bridge any stronger?

Nonvertebral fractures increase 300 to 600 percent in patients undergoing fluoride therapy.[6]

Extensive research shows that even a *low* level of fluoridation correlates with higher fracture statistics.[7,8,9]

A report in the *Journal of the American Medical Association*, 1992, shows that a significant increase in hip fractures in men and women over 65 occurs in Brigham City, Utah, where the water is fluoridated at 1 part per million (the assumed safe level) when compared with two other cities in

Utah which have only 0.3 parts per million. This is the fourth report of an ecological link between fluoridated water and an extended incidence of hip fractures published in the last two years.[10]

Based on all this information, if you live in a city where fluoridation is in use, you should take tap water off the list, too. There's still controversy, unfortunately, about whether fluoridation is a useful strategy for improving the dental health of children. I won't get into that one here, except to report that the gap in the tooth decay rate in children living in fluoridated and nonfluoridated water districts has been narrowing. Studies have found that the divergence has all but disappeared.[11]

Note that no health benefits are claimed for older adults with fluoridated water, and a consensus is developing that *fluoridation can be harmful to the mature population.*

I have never allowed my family to consume fluoridated water when I could control the situation.

One more problem concerning water: *Chlorinated water, especially if consumed on a high fat diet, reduces calcium absorption.*[12] Almost all tap water is chlorinated. If the kitchen faucet MUST be your water source, fill a pitcher with water and let it stand uncovered either in the fridge or at room temperature for 24 hours. Most of the chlorine will evaporate.[13]

Are you concluding that perils lurk at every swallow? How about spring water, perhaps with a twist of lemon or lime to embellish your drink? In most cities you can have good water delivered (like milk in the old days).

Cut Down on Meat

You've heard it again and again, but little attention is paid to this fact: Too much protein causes calcium to be lost in the urine. How much protein do you need? That depends on the *quality* of the protein you are consuming. As a general rule, however, *no more than one and one-half ounces of protein are required for a 150-pound person per day.* That's not a lot, is it? It translates to very little meat or cheese. And even that specified amount is arbitrary.

FIGURE 16

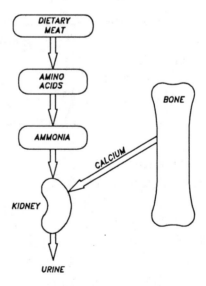

MEAT CONSUMPTION
AND CALCIUM EXCRETION

The excretion of amino acid products from meat often requires additional calcium to be pulled out of bone tissue.

> Things get worse as you get older. Senior meat eaters lose almost twice as much calcium as their vegetarian peers.

No amount of progesterone can compensate totally for calcium loss caused by excessive meat consumption.

A meat-eating animal in the wild balances its calcium deficiency and phosphorus excess by consuming bones. Any veterinarian will confirm that when dogs are fed leftover hamburger or commercially-prepared all-meat dog food, skeletal disease is the consequence.

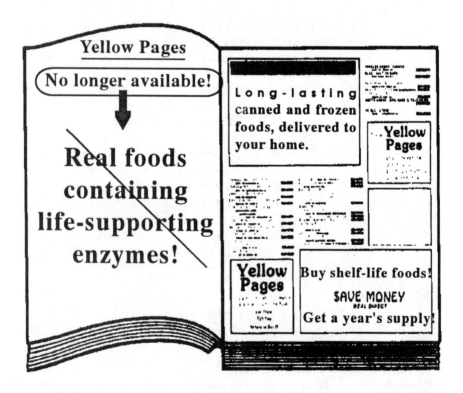

MEMOS

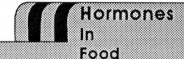

Hormones In Food

ABSTRACT: In the absence of effective federal regulation, the meat industry uses hundreds of animal-feed additives, including antibiotics, tranquilizers, pesticides, animal drugs, artificial flavors, industrial wastes, and *growth-promoting hormones*, with little or no concern about the carcinogenic and other toxic effects of dietary residues of these additives. Illustratively, after decades of misleading assurances of the safety of diethylstilbestrol (DES) and its use as a growth-promoting animal-feed additive, the United States finally banned its use in 1979, some 40 years after it was first shown to be carcinogenic. The meat industry then promptly switched to other carcinogenic additives, particularly the natural sex hormones estradiol, progesterone, and testosterone, which are implanted in the ears of more than 90 percent of commercially raised feedlot cattle. Unlike the synthetic DES, residues of which can be monitored and use of which was conditional on a seven-day preslaughter withdrawal period, residues of natural hormones are not detectable, since they cannot be practically differentiated from the same hormones produced by the body. The relationship between recently increasing cancer rates and the lifetime exposure of the U.S. population to dietary residues of these and other unlabeled carcinogenic feed additives is a matter of critical public health concern.

Epstein SS. The chemical jungle: today's beef industry. *International Journal of Health Services*, 1990, 20(2):277-80.

Reduce Phosphorus Intake

Recall that phosphorus is an integral part of bone material but that too much is not in your best health interest. It's the *proportion* of phosphorus to calcium that's significant. In the presence of too much phosphorus, hormonal feedback mechanisms can block the proper assimilation of phosphorus *and* calcium.[14] The average American diet, high in phosphorus, just doesn't contain the recommended one-to-one calcium/phosphorus ratio.

So even though cheese (unlike meat) contains calcium, the amount of calcium is no match for the phosphorus content. Consuming high calcium foods like milk doesn't serve to correct the problem or alter the ratio. Here's one reason why: Milk and milk products are almost equal sources of both phosphorus and calcium but sometimes contain even more phosphorus. (Cottage cheese is an example—it has considerably more phosphorus than calcium.) At higher levels of ingestion, calcium absorption decreases sharply. You are an efficient calcium picker-upper only when calcium is present at low levels.

> Even if the *same* quantities of calcium and phosphorus are consumed (as in milk and many milk products), the absorption ratio shifts so that more phosphorus than calcium gets absorbed, disturbing the health-promoting ratio.

At the risk of repetition, please check Table 4 on the next page for a list of phosphorus-loaded foods.

TABLE 4
HIGH PHOSPHORUS FOODS

➤ Almost all processed or canned meats (hot dogs, ham, bacon)
➤ Processed cheeses
➤ Baked products that include phosphate baking powder (commonly used)
➤ Cola and other soft drinks
➤ Instant soups and puddings
➤ Toppings and seasonings
➤ Breads
➤ Cereals
➤ Meats (meat contains *fifty times* more phosphorus than calcium!)
➤ Potatoes
➤ Phosphate food additives: phosphoric acid, pyrophosphate, polyphosphates, such as chelators, sequestering and emulsifying agents, acidulators, water binders, including sodium phosphate, potassium phosphate, and phosphoric acid

Quite a list, and too bad; it includes foods that I personally don't want to give up (baked potatoes, for example).

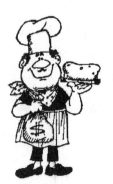

The more processed, the higher the profits.

The food charts can help you to evaluate the phosphorus and calcium content of many popular foods. There are surprises here, too; not all healthful foods are high in calcium, and some have copious amounts of phosphorus! Use the data as a rough guide to gauge your *average* calcium/phosphorus ratio, but don't make a religion of avoiding unprocessed high-phosphorus foods. Those that have not been mushed, mashed, or mangled have other nutritional redeeming features. Soft drinks have none. Real foods—like whole grains and potatoes—do.

Avoid Harmful Packaging

High levels of tin may be found in some processed foods due to the addition of tin-based preservatives and stabilizers, or to corrosion and leaching of the metal from unlacquered cans or from tin foils used in packaging.

Diets including a high proportion of canned vegetables and canned fish could supply amounts of tin in excess of acceptable quantities.

> A variety of adverse effects of tin have been reported, including those on the calcium content of bone.[15]

Packaging and labels can be deceiving. Shop wisely.

Avoid Aluminum in Underarm Spray and in Antacids

Environmental exposure to aluminum is universal and increasing. It is commonly found in food, medicine, and cosmetics. Sources of aluminum are antacids, underarm sprays, aluminum cookware (especially when preparing acid foods such as tomato sauce in these pots), air conditioning (sorry about that), environmental contamination, children's aspirin, some baking powders, many white flours, and foods grown in contaminated soil.

Aluminum from antacids has become a serious problem because it has been shown to be absorbed twenty to thirty times more than occurs normally.[16] Aluminum poisoning and spontaneous fractures are definite associations. Aluminum-induced bone problems may be more widespread than we previously realized.

You can be more selective. Purchase unleaded cans of food, look for aluminum-free sprays and baking powder, and use stainless steel or enamel cookware. Aluminum-free digestive aids are available.

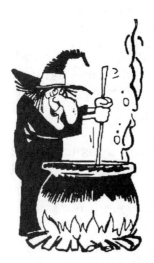

I wonder why I got that subpoena from the FDA demanding to know what additives I use.

Grow Your Own Sprouts

Grow your own sprouts, or at least buy them and eat them. They are a good source of absorbable calcium, and are low in phosphorus. Sprouts are likely to be the only truly fresh food to which you have access—living and growing right up to the moment they enter your mouth—a dim reflection of an era when *all* our food was that fresh, and very important for many reasons that don't directly concern us here.

Suffice it to say that you're doing yourself a great disservice if you don't buy sprouts or grow them in your kitchen. Seeds may be consumed at any stage of sprouting, but harvesting at peak offers the most value. Vitamin C is actually synthesized during germination, and the concentrations of some of the B vitamins is also increased, along with other nutrients. Since seeds vary, it's advisable to experiment, using a good sprouting book as a guide. Alfalfa, mung and chickpeas are excellent sprouts for beginners. I purchase already-sprouted sunflower seeds (called sunflower lettuce) and buckwheat. I sprout my own clover, radish, lentil, chickpeas, green peas, wheatberries, mung, azuki, and alfalfa (recall that alfalfa is a phyto-estrogen).

Exercise—Outdoors

There is no controversy when we discuss exercise and the need for natural outdoor exposure. Everyone agrees that moderate weight-bearing exercise stimulates bones to keep them strong.

The bookstores are full of books about aerobic programs, written by people with far more expertise in this area. If you don't already have a reasonable exercise plan, walk to the nearest bookstore— leave your car where it is.

I'll add one note, though. Fast walking is still the best exercise around. It's safe, weight-bearing, relatively low-impact, always available, and you already know how to do it. (As Dr. Lee says, "Walking is good for the bowels, good for circulation, and good for seeing what the neighbors are doing.")

If you want additional back-strengthening strategies, go dancing or check out some of the exercise machines. Excessive activity, however, can inhibit bone growth and gives rise to stress fractures.[17] This occurs because of calcium loss during vigorous exercise.

When you are a seasoned walker, try experimenting with a few different types of motion. Pretend you are the Tin Man in *The Wizard of Oz*. You will walk with muscles more tense, and this will slow you down. Then see yourself as a rag doll, with your whole body loose, arms swinging freely, taking larger strides. This Raggedy Anne or Andy mode is far better.

That exercised bones are less subject to damage is demonstrated by the fact that if you are right-handed, the bones on your left side are more apt to break than those on your right side.[18] A routine of physical activity may be as beneficial for your skeleton as it is for your heart.

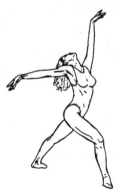

¤

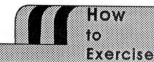

WHY WALKING IS BEST

In addition to its beneficial effects on bone, exercise stimulates hormonal secretions and is capable of creating euphoria more powerful than mood-elevating drugs. Osteoporosis is a nutritional-deficiency disease and the right kind of exercise is an important component of nutrition.

Good exercise is both aerobic and weight-bearing. Golf is weight-bearing, but not aerobic. Swimming is aerobic, but not weight-bearing. Fast walking is the best possible exercise. Aerobic exercises are those that make your heart accelerate for a sustained period of time, causing a need for more air (oxygen). An aerobic exercise is go-go-go and not stop-and-go. A weight-bearing exercise keeps you on your feet.

An exercise session should last for at least twenty minutes. If optimal benefit is the goal, plan your aerobic activity at least five times a week.

A regular outdoor walking schedule guarantees that both your body and eyes will be exposed to daylight. This causes an increased output of various glandular secretions, to say nothing of promoting absorption of the priceless vitamin D, the power substance for the prevention of osteoporosis.

No matter how old you are or what level of activity you participated in before starting, fitness can be achieved with continuous vigorous walking for regular periods of time each day. (You see, there are no excuses.)

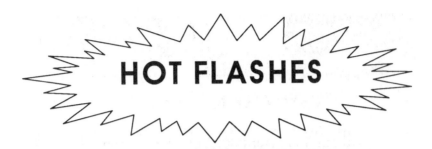

HOT FLASHES

➤ More than two and one-half cups of coffee a day significantly increases the risk of hip fracture in menopausal women.
American Journal of Epidemiology, 1990[19]

➤ Caffeine (from coffee, tea, and/or soda) stimulates the release of calcium from bone.
Calcified Tissue International, 1992[20]

➤ Vegetarians' diets have a somewhat higher nutrient density for folate, thiamin, vitamin C, and vitamin A.
American Journal of Clinical Nutrition, 1988[21]

➤ Vegetarians' diets contain less total fat, saturated fatty acids, and cholesterol and higher dietary fiber.
American Journal of Clinical Nutrition, 1988[22]

➤ Studies of 1600 women reveal that those who follow a vegetarian diet for at least 20 years have only an 18-percent bone mineral loss by age 80, whereas meat eaters have 35-percent less bone mineral.
American Journal of Clinical Nutrition, 1988[23]

➢ Although there is a gain in bone density from fluoride ingestion, it increases fracture risk.

> *Revue du Rhumatisme et des Maladies Osteo-Articulaires*, 1992[24]

➢ Sodium fluoride cannot be recommended for routine use at this time.

> *PostGraduate Medicine*, 1990[25]

➢ Preservation of bone mass through early premenopausal life can be favored by *good nutrition and physical activity.*

> *Clinical Rheumatology*, 1989; *Osteoporosis International*, 1990[26,27]

➢ Women on oral contraceptives are more susceptible to osteoporosis in later years because of diminished levels of magnesium.

> *American Journal of Clinical Nutrition*, 1964[28]

➢ Athletic women may become amenorrheic if *undernutrition* coexists with increasing exercise loads.

> *Sports Medicine*, 1992[29]

➢ Milk and milk products are among the poorest sources of copper (important in postmenopausal osteoporosis). Lactose, as in dairy products, may interfere with copper metabolism.

> *Medical Hypotheses*, 1988[30]

➢ An exercise-hormone regimen is more effective than exercise and calcium supplementation for increasing bone mass.

> *New England Journal of Medicine*, 1991[31]

~~ ENDNOTES ~~ *The fantasy continues...*

Our fantasy continues to be revealing. Now we see why ice cream won't melt, why grains grow quickly with artificial fertilizer, why peanut butter doesn't have to be mixed, why salt flows freely, why butter doesn't have to be refrigerated, why butter is yellow all year round, why the cream in milk doesn't rise to the top, why potato chips are never soggy, why bread stays soft, why rice doesn't stick to the pot, why rice cooks in a minute, why mashed potatoes come in a box, why all the breaded shrimp pieces are the same size, and why sweet cream—30 days old—is fresh-smelling. Oy! We can even see why tomotoes won't crack when hurled against a wall at 12 miles an hour!

How can we protect ourselves against the toxins we swallow, the polluted air we breathe? How can we put back into our food that which should have been there to begin with? I believe, along with many researchers and clinical practitioners the world over, that part of the answer is the use of supplements.

Webster's
sup.ple.ment
(1) something added to complete a thing;
(2) something added to supply a deficiency.

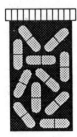

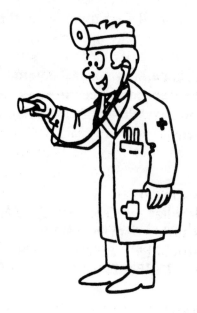

If you continue with quick-fix pudding, instant coffee, jiffy-fast supper and super swift-quick dinners, you can look forward to an early, quick, swift, instant death.

12

SUPPLEMENTS FOR HEALTH

Take Your Vitamins

Vitamin C

If it had been up to me to name vitamins, I would have named this one first. It's hard to find any disorder for which no improvement is shown with the addition of vitamin C. The reason? This nutrient has an incredible number of different roles throughout your body.

Vitamin C is a *water-soluble antioxidant,* which means two things:

(1) It protects complicated proteins from oxidation—that is, destruction that occurs by combining with oxygen.

(2) It is easily carried to and from places needed because it dissolves in water.

Among the lesser-known functions of vitamin C is its role in collagen, the flexible part of your composite bone structure.

Vitamin C helps to repair collagen and to build it up. So an ample supply of vitamin C is important for good bone health. We know just a little about how or why.

How much vitamin C should you take? Everybody's mileage varies, and a dosage couldn't possibly be suggested for you without being familiar with your cellular chemistry. I can say that the recommended daily allowance of only 60 milligrams is far too scant for most of us—either for therapy *or* prevention. That amount is widely acknowledged in the research literature to be unrealistically low.

At the other end of the scale, one doctor has had excellent results with ill patients using therapeutic doses of up to *50 grams* (that's 50,000 milligrams!).[1] High doses are often justified by comparing the amounts of vitamin C synthesized by other mammals having the ability to make their own. During stress, these animals increase their production of vitamin C manyfold. (It is theorized that humans and a few other animals have lost this convenient capability.) On this basis, high doses of vitamin C appear to be reasonable.

Another rationale for taking high doses is that animals manufacture vitamin C in their cells, but we have to swallow it, so some gets lost during digestion.

Overdosing on vitamin C is almost impossible because of how easy it is to determine when you've taken more than you can use. Mild diarrhea is the alarm signal—a quick consequence of exceeding the so-called "bowel-tolerance" level. Eating vitamin C to bowel tolerance means increasing your intake by increments of 100, 250, or even 500 milligrams every week or so—until your stomach reacts. Then you back off to the last comfortable dose, and that amount becomes your daily requirement.

> At times of stress or illness the amount of vitamin C that will cause your stomach to scream back at you is always significantly higher. In other words, you require a lot more vitamin C when you are not up to par.

Personally, I take about four grams (4,000 milligrams) of vitamin C per day, mostly in an esterified form. I require that amount to keep me free of the respiratory problems that plague me whenever I reduce the quantity. I increase the dosage when I am under either physical or emotional stress.

Vitamin D

As so clearly explained in the *Journal of Cellular Biochemistry*, 1992, the main regulator of calcium absorption is vitamin D. This nutrient is manufactured in your skin under the influence of UV-light and is found in limited amounts in just a few foods (egg yolk, certain species of fish, fish liver, and butter). Vitamin D is then converted to more potent forms (or metabolites) in your liver and kidney. With advancing age and skin-cancer scares, men and women tend to have less and less sunlight exposure—the leading natural source of vitamin D.[2]

Among the theories to explain estrogen therapy's effectiveness is one that indicates that estrogen helps the conversion of vitamin D to its active, hormonal form—vitamin D_3.

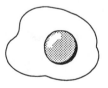

Egg yolks are a good source of vitamin D.

A deficiency of vitamin D is all it takes to develop seriously unhealthy bones. Despite the fact that milk and other foods are routinely fortified with vitamin D, even healthy older people are normally found to be vitamin-D deficient.

The best insurance against vitamin D deficiency is to spend more time in the sunlight, where the vitamin D is free! A 30-minute sun-bath should provide 300 to 350 units.[3] An hour is even better, but if a half hour of time in the sun is not possible, the amount of vitamin D_3 found in a good multi-vitamin supplement should be sufficient.

Keep in mind that vitamin D absorption diminishes with age. (Lucky are those of us who grew up on cod-liver oil. Today, emulsified cod-liver oil is a good supplemental source of vitamin D.)

Adequate levels of vitamin D can help prevent osteoporosis in both women *and* men.[4]

When you look at the metabolic pathways involved for vitamin D—from the sun or food to bone formation—you can understand why researchers refer to osteoporosis as a disease of the liver and kidneys! (See Figure 17 on page 163.)

Boron and magnesium, among other minerals, also have roles to play in vitamin D utilization. Perhaps that's why these nutrients are crucial to bone health. (See the sections on these minerals later in this chapter.)

FIGURE 17

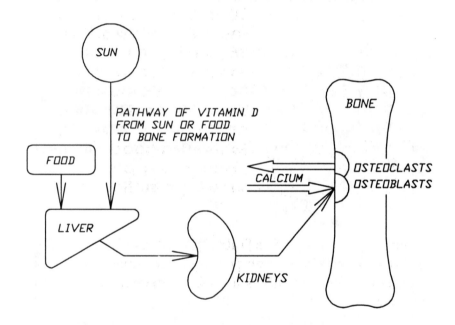

VITAMIN D FROM SOURCE TO BONE

For calcium to be incorporated into your bone structure, vitamin D is a necessity. But this nutrient is provided by only a limited number of foods and by sunlight exposure.

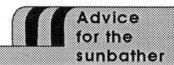

WORSHIP THE SUN—
JUST A LITTLE

Don't be chased into the shade 100 percent of the time by skin-cancer warnings. Skin cancer comes from your body's lack of antioxidants to cope with overexposure. Limited exposure, up to one hour a day, can improve your status on the health/illness scale.

Just don't forget your antioxidants. Antioxidants such as:

> ➤ vitamin A
> ➤ beta-carotene
> ➤ vitamin C
> ➤ vitamin E
> ➤ and selenium

help escort toxins right out of your system in the presence of healthy metabolism.

(As my ten-year-old grandson said when he learned about antioxidants, "Oh, so it's not my A-B-C's I have to pay attention to, but my A-C-E's.")

Vitamin A & Beta-Carotene

Vitamin A is particularly essential for maintaining the integrity of your intestinal walls so they can absorb nutrients (like calcium) with optimal efficiency. Vitamin A and more specifically its precursor, *beta-carotene,* have been shown to provide a very measurable protective effect against many types of cancer. While vitamin A itself is fat-soluble and can be toxic in extremely high doses, beta-carotene is water soluble and is a much safer nutritional supplement. Nearly every cell can convert beta-carotene to vitamin A as needed—provided your thyroid is in good functioning shape and that you have enough zinc—among other lesser-known relationships.

> The enzyme that converts beta-carotene to vitamin A uses zinc.

Vitamin A and beta-carotene are found in ample quantities in yellow and deep green vegetables and in fruit. A large raw carrot, for example, contains 11,000 international units. Dr. Lee, along with most other nutrition-oriented physicians, suggests 25,000 international units per day as a reasonable supplement.[5]

My personal approach is to keep plenty of fresh carrots on hand (organic when available), and these, together with sprouts, are my most frequently-eaten basic snack. I save most of the beta-carotene supplements for the days when I can't eat at least a carrot or two along with handfuls of sunflower "lettuce" and/or other green sprouts.

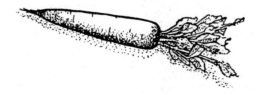

Vitamin E

One reason why vitamin E is often recommended by physicians who specialize in treating women is because this nutrient plays a role in the production and metabolism of sex hormones.

Vitamin E can enhance the utilization of estrogen stores in your adrenal or fat tissues.[6]

Vitamin E also helps to alleviate breast tenderness. In fact, vitamin E deficiency is associated with breast cancer. It has also been shown to slow the process of skin wrinkling and to protect bone marrow from toxicity.[7,8]

For PMS victims, vitamin E is related to the interactions in the multiple biochemical conversions that lead to prostaglandin production. (Note how so many of the nutrients that help to alleviate PMS also help to mitigate menopause symptoms.)

In addition to taking a vitamin E supplement, here's another way to add vitamin E on a daily basis. Soak a tablespoon of wheatberries for 8 to 12 hours, then rinse and sprout the seeds for about two days. This is an inexpensive way to get wheat germ oil (which is extracted commercially from the germ of the wheat) and fiber (taken from the outer coat of the seed). The sprouted wheatberries are sweet and crunchy. They're great in salads or just as is.

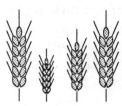 Sprouted wheatberry seeds are chock full of natural vitamin E and have a high fiber content.

Take Your Minerals

Silicon

Did you know that silicon is the second most abundant element on earth, second only to oxygen? Silicon is as plentiful as sand on the beach—literally! Yet this substance has enormous capacity to turn degenerative processes of aging and disease into regenerative processes of healing and vitality. Silicon is so universal in biological function—and so common in our environment—that it is taken for granted.

> Despite its abundance, our diets are seriously silicon-deficient.

When food is processed, fiber is usually the first to go, and silicon disappears with it. Stripped cereals and other treated foods have reduced our supplies of this valuable mineral.

Silicon plays its most conspicuous role in calcium metabolism. A mounting body of evidence points to organic vegetable silicon as one of the key factors in the control of osteoporosis.

It has been conjectured that people in other countries who have no bone disorders despite not getting enough calcium (by our standards) are probably consuming adequate amounts of silicon.[9]

With the exception of mother's milk, silicon levels tend to be higher in plant foods than in foods from animal sources. Foods highest in silicon include grains—especially oats, barley, and the fiber part of brown rice.[10,11] Silicon is also found in many fruits and vegetables (as tabulated in the Food Tables).

The herb *equisetum*, commonly known as *horsetail*, is a particularly good source of silicon. Horsetail is a wayside weed that grows nearly everywhere. It's one of those ancient herbs, used for millennia. Horsetail tea, for example, has long been recommended for the regeneration of fingernails. I have been an advocate of horsetail extract for decades.

Note that *silicone*, ending with an "e," usually refers to an inorganic form of the mineral which is not useful for bone health. The best sources of dietary organic silicon, by far, are those mentioned above.

Boron

A mineral that offers the same benefits as estrogen replacement therapy without the side effects? Yes! In 1986, the consequences of major mineral metabolism in postmenopausal women were examined by the United States Department of Agriculture. It was found that boron supplementation markedly reduces the urinary excretion of calcium and magnesium.

Blood levels of estrogen in those taking boron rise to levels found in women on estrogen replacement therapy.

When we think of bone as the main storage site for boron, as well as for calcium, the puzzle pieces begin to fit together.

ERT ▷ ESTROGEN ▷ SIDE EFFECTS

BORON ▷ ESTROGEN ▷ NO SIDE EFFECTS

Boron is vital for the production of the active form of vitamin D and possibly for estrogen as well. F. Nielson, Ph.D., the nutritionist who conducted the research for the United States Department of Agriculture, believes that boron's favorable effect on the balance of hormones dramatically improves calcium retention. Additional studies reported in the *Journal of Trace Elements and Experimental Medicine* in 1992 confirm that boron enhances and mimics some effects of estrogen ingestion in postmenopausal women.[12]

Can we get enough boron from our foods? Not usually, according to reports in the *American Dietetic Association,* 1991. Excessive use of soluble chemical fertilizers has damaged the soils, and low concentrations of minerals affect several aspects of mineral metabolism. Levels of boron in this country have dropped considerably in the last 50 years.[13]

Alfalfa and kelp (also high in silicon) are excellent sources of boron. Under ideal growing conditions, spinach and snap beans contain significant quantities. Cabbage, lettuce, apples, leafy greens, legumes, and musk-melon leaves are next in line. But you would have to eat about five apples or fourteen pounds of lettuce to get the necessary three milligrams of boron. The Food Tables list the ranges of boron concentrations typically found in some foods. Note the wide variation. A lot depends on the soil and water conditions that prevailed where and when the food was grown. (For more information on osteoporosis and bone health, refer to my booklet, *Startling New Facts About Osteoporosis.*)

Another government study shows that people have fewer cavities in areas where water contains boron and other trace minerals. These same elements found in abundance in cavity-free regions are sorely lacking in neighborhoods prone to a greater percentage of tooth decay.

Magnesium

Healthy bone is comprised of 20 percent calcium, but only 0.1 percent magnesium. Small as that amount is, magnesium plays an important role in converting vitamin D to its active form. Magnesium is also a powerful agent in the fixation of calcium.

High phosphorus levels in your diet can aggravate the symptoms of a magnesium deficiency.

You can see how this business of nutrient dependency and bone health gets to be as fragile as a house of cards. Too much phosphorus affects magnesium, which affects vitamin D conversion, which affects calcium absorption, which affects bone health. And that's just one of many complex conditional pathways.

While the typical North American diet is deficient in magnesium, blood serum levels may be normal due to self-regulating mechanisms that keep these levels up *at the expense of cellular magnesium.* So the best test for magnesium content is one that measures its level in your red blood cells.

Foods which have significant quantities of magnesium include eggs, liver, leafy greens, whole grains, legumes, seeds, almonds, black-eyed peas, curry, and mustard powder.

Stop for a moment and think about whether or not you have included any of these foods in your meals in the last few days. The leafy-green category does *not* include iceberg lettuce; the whole-grain category does *not* include cold, boxed cereals or white rice; and, obviously, curry and mustard powder would *not* be consumed in enough quantity to make a difference. Morning eggs (certified organic) and a handful of sprouted lentils usually help to assure my daily magnesium fix. I supplement on other days.

Potassium

As already mentioned, the sodium-potassium pump that manages every cell in your body also impacts on premenstrual bloating. Part of the reason that Asian women don't have our female afflictions may be their rich diets of dulse, kelp, and soybeans, which contain far more potassium than most other food substances. (For example, dulse, a seaweed, has 8,060 milligrams of potassium in 100 grams; a banana contains 370.)

Because our diets of processed foods disturb the natural ratios of sodium and potassium and because it is virtually impossible to get enough potassium in our usual food supply to counter the sodium content of our foods, *even if we try*, I recommend well-designed potassium supplementation. (My preference is the liquid tonic preparations that have small amounts of various herbs and other whole-food-based nutrients added to the potassium.)

Meanwhile, parsley, spinach, and asparagus are good foods of choice to add to your meals around "bloating" time. My book, *Everything You Always Wanted to Know About Potassium But Were Too Tired to Ask,* answers many of the specific questions about potassium metabolism.

Chromium

Why do 98.5 percent of most European people over the age of 50 have enough chromium, when only about one in four Americans in that same age category do not? As for the rest of our population, short supplies of chromium subject almost every one of us to many problems, both subtle and serious. Too bad our American food supply has detached itself from nature.

Impaired glucose tolerance, high levels of circulating insulin, and insulin resistance are common dilemmas among contraceptive pill users and menopausal women.[14] Since chromium improves glucose tolerance and makes insulin more effective, this mineral may be an excellent addition. (See Table 5 below.)

TABLE 5
SIGNS OF CHROMIUM DEFICIENCY

Chromium (200 micrograms daily) in the niacin-bound form, *chromium polynicotinate*, can be helpful if:

➤ you cannot lose weight.
➤ you are under stress.
➤ you overreact to ordinary circumstances.
➤ you participate in athletics or aerobics.
➤ you have any problems with blood-sugar metabolism (too high or too low).
➤ you sustain elevated cholesterol.
➤ you just want to insure your good health.
➤ you are tired too often.

Most of all, chromium polynicotinate can help to maximize energy potential.[15]

Zinc

Our appreciation for the importance of zinc becomes more pronounced with each research paper. All the carrots in the world would be useless for the many functions requiring vitamin A in the absence of sufficient *zinc*. Zinc helps to transform beta-carotene into usable vitamin A.

> Perhaps it's not just an old wives' tale that oysters are especially good for your sex life—oysters are a rich source of zinc!

Consider Other Supplements

Hydrochloric Acid

Hydrochloric acid has already been cited as essential for bone/calcium metabolism. The least costly way to determine if you are deficient in hydrochloric acid is to purchase some in supplemental form at the health store. If you find after taking it that you can digest a food that formerly caused difficulty (pork chops, for example—if you still eat fatty meats), you can probably confirm your deficiency. A more accurate way is to consult your physician for scientific testing. You might point out to your physician that you are interested in your hydrochloric acid status because YOU KNOW that hydrochloric acid is necessary for good bone metabolism.

Gamma Linolenic Acid (GLA)

Essential fatty acids are just that—*essential*. They are important not only because they are a major component of the membranes surrounding all cells, but also because they help form substances known as *prostaglandins*.

One of the most powerful unsaturated fatty acids is *gamma linolenic acid* (GLA). GLA is found in very few foods and can only be manufactured in your body through a complex series of metabolic processes—*which decline in efficiency with age.* In fact, most people have difficulty converting polyunsaturated oils to this activated form. Yet GLA is critical for the production of good-guy prostaglandins, which play a role in bone formation. Prostaglandins are at the door of *every* cell, orchestrating many vital metabolic functions.[16]

Fortunately, GLA is available in supplemental form. Sources of GLA are the oils of the seeds of black currants, borage, and primrose.

Are you recognizing a pattern here? Many of these nutrients seem to come from various fresh, natural foods or food sources. Eat with one nutrient in mind, and odds are you'll be supplying most of the others without any additional attention. It shouldn't come as any surprise that vegetarians (the *nutrient*-oriented type, not the *Twinkies* people) have higher bone density than age-matched meat eaters.

This is far from a complete list of the vitamins, minerals, and trace elements that are important for avoiding the problems addressed here. Vitamin B_6 deficiency, for example, is critically important in osteoporosis and may also play a key role in preventing arteriosclerosis and heart disease.

B_6 gets good grades from those who suffer from PMS—perhaps because it helps depression and fluid retention. *It also stimulates the production of progesterone.*

Then there's manganese, copper, and strontium (nonradio-active, of course!). But if your diet is heavily biased toward fresh and unprocessed foods and if you're paying attention to possible deficiencies that call for supplementation, it's unlikely that you'll miss *any* of the significant substances, not even those that are more obscure. A carefully selected quality multi-vitamin/mineral supplement plus a few supplements discussed in the following pages should help to cover all bases. But please don't think of your supplements as a permanent replacement for a good diet!

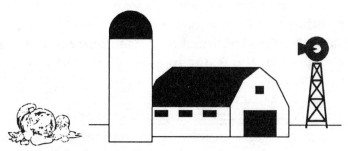

Whole foods are not mushed, mashed or mangled, and are the least harmful.

Select a Few Food-Type Supplements

I have always been a strong advocate of food-based supplementation because these products run the gamut: they contain nutrients already identified and those yet to be discovered. More than that, they come in a more natural matrix, so that nutrients designed to "go together" are all present at roll call. Although by no means a complete list, garlic, acidophilus, flaxseed oil, beet crystals, kamut grass extract, and bee pollen are among those I like to recommend. I take several of these every day, varying my selection from time to time. Starting with garlic, here's why:

Garlic

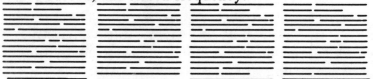

EXTRA!!! The Times EXTRA!!!

GARLIC EXTRACT CURES CANCER
IN TEST ANIMALS

Groups of hamsters were treated for up to fourteen weeks with a topical carcinogen. Prior to, during, and after treatment the test animals were also treated with a solution of an active ingredient found in garlic. The result? A significant reduction in tumor frequency, tumor burden, and lesion frequency.[17]

Wait! There's more.

EXTRA!!! The Times EXTRA!!!

GARLIC PROTECTS AGAINST
MAMMARY TUMORS

A study determined the influence of supplemental garlic powder on induced mammary tumors. Although food intake and weight gain were not influenced, the garlic powder significantly delayed the onset of tumors and reduced the total mammary tumor incidence. Consumption of garlic powder also significantly depressed the binding of the carcinogen to mammary cell DNA.[18]

These recent studies scientifically confirm what the wisdom of the ages has known for a long time. Garlic has been used as a preventive and therapeutic agent for millennia (Sanskrit records document its use 5,000 years ago), perhaps because garlic's antimicrobial properties have been effective against a broad spectrum of bacteria, viruses, and fungi.

If you enjoy war stories about the use of special healing agents, note these about garlic: British soldiers applied garlic water directly to wounds during World War I; the Russians used garlic both internally and externally to speed healing during World War II.[19]

Deodorized forms of garlic may work as well as pure unadulterated fresh garlic. Probably the most important constituent of garlic is a chemical called *allicin*, the sulphurous and smelly substance that also seems to give garlic most of its outstanding medicinal qualities. Allicin is a natural antibiotic—it has even been compared favorably with penicillin for the treatment of certain classes of infections. But allicin in its active form is relatively scarce in fresh garlic. Its precursor, *alliin*, must be converted to allicin by the enzyme *allinase*. These two substances do not mix until the garlic is either digested or physically altered—explaining why the garlic smell becomes so strong when garlic is crushed.

A quality supplement is comprised of garlic that has gone through a long-term natural cold-aging process. The alliin is converted to beneficial sulfur compounds and the final product is odorless. The antimicrobial mechanisms of garlic supplements explain some of its effects. One study shows how garlic supplements increase natural immunity through its promotion of killer-cell activity. And test animals given this elixir are better able to resist the flu! The successful merging of traditional observation with high technology is something to be respected.

Flaxseed oil

I like to tell the flaxseed oil story, so get ready for a little food history.

Once upon a time, every town and hamlet had its own oil mill. Many plants and seeds were used, but the favorite for producing oil was the flaxseed. It had a nutty, rich, almost creamy flavor, which (according to legend) tasted a lot like fresh butter.

As hamlets grew to towns and towns to cities, it became common-place to have fresh oil delivered door-to-door, just like milk, eggs, and butter at a later time. Flaxseed oil was sold in small quantities and used only if fresh—the people understood just how its health-sustaining and therapeutic values worked best!

But oil-making practices changed with the use of machinery and specialization—efforts which made daily chores less arduous. Small presses were replaced with automated continuous-feed inventions. These were run at rates and pressures that raised the temperature of the oil far above the boiling point. Hydrocarbon solvents extracted more flax oil at a faster rate. The oil was also bleached, de-gummed, and deodorized. Heat, light, air and time provoked rancidity. So flaxseed oil, because it was no longer a "pure" and health-promoting product, eventually disappeared from the marketplace, taken over by corn and soy oil, among others.

As we gained knowledge, we learned that fresh flaxseed oil contained two fatty acids that the human body couldn't make: *linoleic acid* (LA) and *linolenic acid* (LNA). The only way to get these fatty acids is to eat them. That's why they are called *essential*.

We also learned that LA and LNA are precursors—or chemical building blocks of a whole class of more elaborate fatty acids. These, in turn, are building blocks of literally thousands of enzymes, hormones, and prostaglandins—having to do with many cellular functions, including bone formation. Arachidonic acid, made from LA, regulates viral infection and resistance to toxins. Derivatives of LNA reduce the risk of fatal heart attacks and help to manufacture substances which control and limit blood platelet aggregation (the sticking-together of blood platelets).

> Flaxseed oil has a slow absorption rate, and is high in magnesium (necessary for vitamin D conversion, as cited above), rich in lecithin, and unmatched in its percentage as a natural source of omega 3's. *Flaxseed oil has the components needed for good prostaglandin metabolism.*

An ample supply of LA and LNA is another way of insuring sufficient supplies of health-promoting nutrients—provided in abundance by fresh flaxseed oil. But what about the rancidity problems? Shelf-life? Over-processing? All the detrimental effects of this century's current and careless foodways habits?

Good news! It's BACK TO THE FUTURE: Today, you *can* get *pure, organic, unadulterated, non-rancid flaxseed oil* —in protective capsules—to add to your supplement regime. (Be sure to refrigerate.)

Red Beet Crystals

The rich, sweet, pungent red root of the beet is a wizard's brew of vitamins, minerals, and other important nutrients. I am especially fond of this supplement because it can disguise the taste of not-so-pleasant-tasting liquid nutrient blends.

Beets really are *good for your blood*— a statement assumed to be mythical, deriving from the blood-red color of its juice. Although our mothers and grandmothers couldn't possibly have known the scientific facts, there is something to the legend.

One of the problems with beets is that they require a lot of cooking. Vitamin B_6, so critical to most of the beneficial actions of the nutrients in beets, is sensitive to high temperatures. Since beets are usually boiled for anywhere from thirty minutes to two hours (at 212 degrees F), it's safe to say that a large portion of the original B_6 has departed as a result of the cooking process. Canned beets are subjected to even higher temperatures.

Crystallized beets, dissolved in water, capture the sweetness of beets and make potent nutrient mixtures delightfully palatable—without the losses incurred in the cooking process.

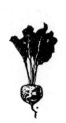 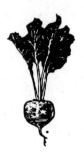 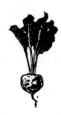

Pollen

Pollen is the male seed of flowers, and, like any seed, it contains across-the-board nutrients. Each pollen grain has from 1,000,000 to 5,000,000 pollen spores, all capable of reproducing the species.

This golden dust is comprised of thousands of enzymes and coenzymes—*many times more than in any other food.* An enzyme is a kind of catalyst, a substance that facilitates or promotes a chemical reaction, but is not itself consumed by the reaction. Enzymes can only be processed by a living organism.

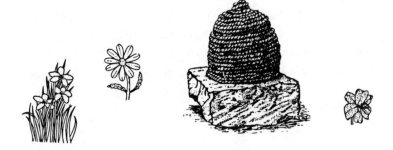

Dong Quai

Dr. Milner recommends *dong quai* (the herb *angelica*) because it is helpful for progesterone metabolism.[20] Dong quai also serves as a pain and allergy reliever—its effectiveness is almost twice that of aspirin. (Dr. Milner also recommends folic acid to protect against deficiencies that may arise with the use of synthetic hormone therapy.)

Cautions:
* Dong quai should not be taken during pregnancy or for excessive menstrual flow.
* Vitamin E and folic acid in high doses should be regulated by your physician.

Kamut

You are probably aware of the "green" revolution in food supplements. Because we have come to realize that young plants are powerful life forms containing high levels of nutrients necessary for good health, the extracts from these shoots are gaining in popularity. Even more digestible than veggies (which are composed mainly of cellulose), young cereal grasses provide readily available vitamins, minerals, and enzymes.

I am always intrigued by the rediscovery of ancient, nutritious foods. The newest and most unique green food supplement available is *green kamut*. Green *what?* Kamut (pronounced ka-moot) is a grain whose history goes back to the cradle of civilization. According to folk lore, seeds discovered in an Egyptian pyramid germinated and sprouted into products bearing a bounty of nutrients. Although this story cannot be confirmed, the specialness of the product and one's imagination make it fun to think that there might just be at least a thread of truth in this tale.

A rich buttery flavor is among kamut's notable properties. An ancestor of our modern durum wheat, kamut is grown organically without having been subjected to the toxins and mutations of today's popular grains. Kamut has demonstrated its superiority in being less allergenic than other more familiar wheat products. Higher in protein, beta-carotene, and chlorophyll, kamut sounds like a new staff of life, doesn't it?

Acidophilus

What? Add more bacteria to your gut? Yes, the good-guy variety, to crowd out bacteria of disreputable lineage. You can resist enemy invasion by entrenching your normal flora with healthful sentries. The easiest way to provide a settlement of proper bacteria is with acidophilus. A good acidophilus supplement loads a few billion acidophilus organisms per gram. The acidophilus bacteria set up housekeeping in your intestine, creating an ecological system that helps to absorb nutrients and create new ones.

Acidophilus is available in a milk base, or vegetarian-grown. A similar helpful bacterium (*lactobacillus bulgaricus*, perhaps a second cousin once removed) is found in *viable* yogurt. (Note the emphasis on viable; not all supermarket yogurts are "live." Health store proprietors can direct you to the "good" yogurt.)

Your great-grandmother produced another equally beneficial strain by "clabbering," or souring, milk in her kitchen. Nearly every healthy society consumed a fermented or cultured food product of one type or another because empirical observation showed that the addition of these foods was associated with good health. According to conclusions of an international medical symposium, such products are of importance in the nutrition of people everywhere—especially in today's world. Fermentation is one of the most important functions of the colonic flora.

There are more living entities in your flora than there are cells in your whole body. Acidophilus contributes favorably to your microflora, performing a wide variety of important functions in nutrition, immunology, and metabolism in general.

Long ago, the process was initiated by organisms present in raw foods, in the air, or on utensils. Today we use specific starter cultures and precise conditions of time and temperature, insuring superior products and microbial safety.

Chinese Medicine

Herbal medicines can also be useful to help you journey through menopause in a more comfortable and self-empowered manner. At best, you can make educated choices about using herbs to improve health as well as for reducing common menopausal symptoms. See the section on page 247 for an account of helpful Chinese herbal medicine prepared by Dr. Herb Kandel.

¤

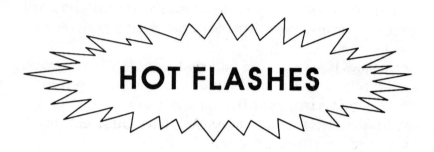

HOT FLASHES

➤ Multivitamin and mineral supplements containing a broad range of vitamins (A, B-2, B-5, B-6, B-9, E) and minerals (Cr, Cu, Mg, Se, Si, Zn) appear to be justified for menopausal women.[21]

Revue Francaise de Gynecologie et D.Obstetrique, 1990

➤ Complete multi's work better for protecting bone marrow cells which have been exposed to carcinogenic and genetic hazards than vitamin C alone.

Mutation Research, 1992[22]

➤ Vitamin C is required for connective tissues such as cartilage and bone.

Nutrition Reviews, 1992[23]

➤ Vitamin C, when administered concurrently with a pesticide, decreases the frequency of the pesticide-induced changes in bone marrow.

Mutation Research, 1993[24]

➤ Vitamin C increases collagen synthesis, and thus, inhibits cancer cell metabolism and proliferation.

Experimental and Toxicologic Pathology, 1992[25]

➤ Test animals given a substance that usually causes bone cells to fragment are protected by vitamin C.

Food and Chemical Toxicology, 1992[26]

➤ The collagen matrix produced by ascorbic acid-treated cells provides the best environment for development.

Nutrition Reviews, 1992[27]

➤ Vitamin C improves bone deformities associated with displaced fractures.

Laboratory Animal Care, 1992[28]

➤ Calcium absorption may be impaired because of a decrease in the ability of the kidneys to produce hormonal vitamin D.

Annual Review of Nutrition, 1990[29]

➤ Decreased bone mineral content is prevalent in infants whose mothers were calcium- and magnesium-deficient during pregnancy.

American College of Nutrition, 1992[30]

➤ Calcium excretion is nutrition-dependent and is influenced by vitamin D status.

Minerva Medica, 1992[31]

➤ Vitamin D influences bone density in middle-aged women.

British Medical Journal, 1992[32]

➤ The active vitamin D component is essential for calcium absorption and bone health.

Journal of Internal Medicine, 1992[33]

➤ Boron is relatively non-toxic.
> *Archives of Environmental Contamination and Toxicology*, 1990[34]

➤ One sign of boron deprivation is depressed bone magnesium.
> *Biological Trace Element Research*, 1988[35]

➤ Boron is important for optimal calcium and, thus, bone metabolism.
> *Biological Trace Element Research*, 1990[36]

➤ Dietary lack of boron and silicon may result in suboptimal function and composition of bone and brain.
> *Asociacion Medica de Puerto Rico*, 1991[37]

➤ Boron deficiency may cause arthritis.
> *Nutrition and Health*, 1991[38]

➤ Magnesium depletion leads to calcium deficiency in the blood.
> *Magnesium Research*, 1992[39]

➤ Magnesium plays a major role in bone formation.
> *American Journal of Clinical Nutrition*, 1964[40]

➤ Silicon is essential for the metabolism of connective and bone tissue.
> *Clinical Therapeutics*, 1991[41]

➤ Silicon is a major constituent of the cells concerned with bone growth.
> *Science of the Total Environment*, 1988[42]

~~ ENDNOTES ~~ *The fantasy continues...*

Throughout these pages, I have used the words *complicated* and *complex* time and again. As our fantasy continues, we can see why: The interrelationships of metabolic processes are more than overwhelming—one nutrient is dependent on another, which is conditional to another, subservient to yet another; one hormone influencing another, and so on.

Now we see how our thyroid and steroid hormones are related. Much more than kissing cousins, they are part of a multi-tiered puppet show. The pituitary pulls the thyroid strings while the thyroid, a pinkish "bow tie" sitting on our windpipe, pulls the bone-growth strings. We watch, as our thyroid dances to the pituitary's tune, producing hormones to deposit or reduce calcium in our bones or in our blood.

Now the act changes. We see the master puppeteer, the hypothalamus, pulling the strings of the pituitary. We watch as a surge of events crashes through our body—*the immediate physical reactions to stress.*

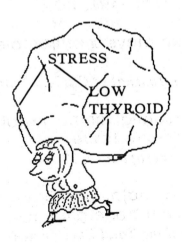

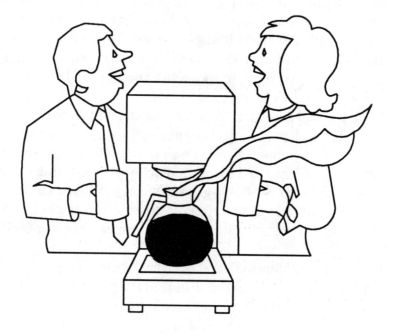

"We emptied the fridge of all the junk food last night. Now there's nothing left but the light bulb. "

13

THE THYROID
AND STRESS CONNECTIONS

THE THYROID CONNECTION

The head bone *is* connected to the neck bone—a concept clearly demonstrated by the association between thyroid function and seemingly separate metabolic actions. It's no news that there is a direct correlation between your immune responses and thyroid function. But important ties also exist between thyroid function and sex hormones,[1] between thyroid hormone and progesterone receptor levels,[2] and between thyroid performance and bone metabolism.[3] And that's just the beginning.

For our purposes, we need to know that low thyroid hormone translates to poor progesterone management, which translates to poor menstrual and menopausal management! Women with low thyroid hormone, for example, invariably have low levels of progesterone in the luteal phase.

Thyroid hormone interacts with FSH (the follicle-stimulating hormone). So an adequate circulating level of thyroid hormone is one of the factors responsible for successful induction of ovulation.[4] The growth of the mammary gland is also regulated by a complex interaction of thyroid and steroid hormones.[5]

> The frequent occurrence of spont-
> aneous abortion in early pregnancy
> may be caused by inadequate thyroid
> hormone.[6]

How do you know if low thyroid function is your problem? Not easily. Frustration about the nonspecific clinical manifestations of a low thyroid output and confusion about the many tests to check for this disorder are commonplace.[7] Signs and symptoms of thyroid deficiency and interpretation of thyroid tests become even more difficult as we get older. As we age, we are more likely to develop problems with fluid and electrolyte balances (more of what we *don't* need at menopause!), which are tied in with thyroid function. A decreased sensitivity of the thirst mechanism may be an important contributor to these imbalances.[8]

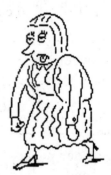

Fatigue may be an indication of a low-functioning thyroid. For symptom-free menstruation and menopausal integrity, thyroid function must be optimal.

One good indication of low thyroid outlay is *cold intolerance*—cold hands and feet. Other benchmarks are tendency to weight gain, dry skin, brittle nails, chronic fatigue, and even constipation. The best indication, however, is to test your pituitary hormone levels rather than your thyroid secretions. Here's why:

Thyroid-stimulating hormone (TSH) is secreted by your pituitary. Very simply, if you require more thyroid hormone, your brain signals your pituitary, which then signals your thyroid to produce more thyroid hormone. So if you have a high TSH, your pituitary is giving your thyroid the message to produce more thyroid hormone. A low TSH is an indication that your thyroid is attempting to close down; it's overproducing. But here's the rub: you may have low TSH as the result of taking an excess of thyroid hormone, prescribed because you had a low thyroid hormone output to begin with! According to researchers reporting in *Postgraduate Medicine*, May 1993, the TSH assay is the single most important test in the diagnosis and treatment of hypothyroidism (low thyroid production).[9]

Because proper thyroid function has such a profound effect on so many organ systems, physicians often prescribe medication for producers of low thyroid hormone. So treatment, if not watched carefully, can be a double-edged sword.

Too much thyroid hormone increases bone turnover, which, in turn, may lead to bone loss from your spine and hip.[10]

Studies have shown that treatment of a low thyroid condition results in loss of cortical and trabecular bone, placing you at risk for osteoporosis.[11,12] The effect of thyroid therapy on bone mineral density has prompted recommendations to prescribe doses of thyroxine at lower levels.[13] If you are on thyroid hormone therapy, discuss this potential problem with your physician.

M E M O S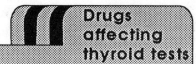

Drugs Affecting Tests
for Determining Thyroid Function

Corticosteroids
   suppress TSH; block conversion of thyroid hormones (T_4 to T_3).

Cough medications
   can induce hypothyroidism if preparation contains iodine.

Estrogens
   falsely increase total T_4 level.

Dilantin
   decreases total T_4 level.

Salicylates (aspirin)
   decrease T_4 level.

You can see how drugs may affect thyroid test results, thereby contributing to misleading conclusions.

MEMOS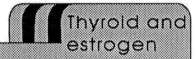

Thyroid Function and Estrogen Activity

One of the thyroid hormones helps to regulate estrogen. Those who are hypothyroid and not secreting enough of this hormone increase the risk of having higher circulating estrogen throughout their bodies.

With a sleepy thyroid, there is a dramatic shift from high to low estrogen at the time of menopause. This extreme shift is apparent in many women who develop osteoporosis. They have trouble making estrogen themselves because of the previously high circulating levels.

Adequate (but not excessive) levels of iodine, zinc, and copper are necessary for the conversion of thyroid hormones.

THE STRESS CONNECTION

> *I suppose I've always been interested in the relation of mind and body, growing up as I did in a culture that separated them distinctly...Every day in this divided world of mind and body, our language betrayed the limitations of our categories. Widow Brown must have died of a broken heart—she never got sick until after her husband was gone.*

So begins the odyssey of Bill Moyers, a respected journalist, as he confirms that mind and body are connected—something the sages have known for centuries. As suggested by the opening statement in his book, *Healing and the Mind*, the concept that thoughts and feelings influence health has often gone by the wayside in our world of specialization.

We are, however, coming closer to understanding some of the "magic" responsible for the mind/body fusion. This connection may be referred to as grandma's insight, but the professionals call it *psychoneuroimmunology*—a coming together of psychology, neurology, and immunology—a kind of therapy that is not old-fashioned but is undeniably old.

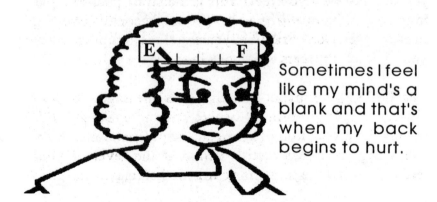

Sometimes I feel like my mind's a blank and that's when my back begins to hurt.

Advances in contemporary medicine have allowed an exploration of the human mind in ways never thought possible before. As explained in *Lancet*, 1993:

> *Many of the functions of the mind, such as perception, learning, speech, memory, sleep and dreams, mood regulation, and pain control are now being understood in terms of physiological and/or biochemical phenomena. Control by the brain over other body functions is known to occur through various processes.*
>
> *Immune cells can secrete substances which in the brain are known to alter sleep, appetite, and hormone secretion.*[14]

Levels of many hormones increase as compensatory reactions. Additional cortisol secretion helps to stabilize blood sugar levels—as occurred, for example, following the Chernobyl accident in response to the radiation exposure. This is just one way our body uses hormones in an attempt to help us adapt to unusual situations.[15]

Can you actually alter hormone metabolism because of how you *think* or how you *feel*? This is a distinct possibility as long as your brain and other body systems continue talking to each other. Don't brain/body interactions take place when you respond with tears while viewing a sad scene in a movie?

Recall that your hypothalamus sends messages to your pituitary, which in turn influences your adrenals and ultimately the production of estrogen and progesterone. Well, stress begins its destructive action at the level of your midbrain—and the target is your hypothalamus.

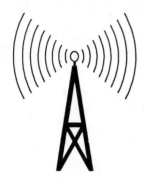

Your hypothalamus works like the dispatching station of a telecommunications center. Once it receives notice of an uncomfortable situation it sends stimulating impulses to its entire territory. This gland is possibly the primary trigger of aging, disease, and health for the whole organism.

We also know that stress affects fatty-acid metabolism, which affects cholesterol, which affects progesterone, which affects cortisol, which affects YOU. This hormonal relay system may be the reason why women report feeling so much better emotionally when they start using natural progesterone.

When your adrenals are overworked (from either emotional *or* physical stress) and can't produce enough of the stress-relieving hormones, your body converts existing progesterone to these hormones. Zap! There goes your progesterone.

If you feel stressed because your mother-in-law is intruding, or because she can't baby-sit tonight, or because your teenager is causing you grief, your calcium may diminish in relation to hormone levels.[16]

So we do know a few facts about how stress relates to PMS and menopausal symptoms. It's not just mind over matter; it's mind *controlling* matter—changing the natural direction of metabolic processes and altering patterns that can be clearly identified.

It has been shown that the combination of stress and junk foods causes women to miss their periods. Take them off the junk food, and the periods come back, even in the presence of the same stress![17] This is in accordance with my belief that *when your stress mechanisms are well nourished they do not break down!* If stress is less destructive under given circumstances, let's work with those particulars, i.e., *better diet.*

As we all know, that's easier said than done. It's very difficult to change your diet and lifestyle. At the very least, consider an alternative such as taking supplements and adding natural progesterone—especially at times of *super* stress. Keep in mind the associations between:

> ➤ destructive stress and junk food

> ➤ destructive stress and lack of nutrients

> ➤ destructive stress and natural progesterone deficiencies

Learning simple stress-relieving mechanisms to help block hurtful events can also be of help. Books and tapes describing such exercises are widely available. Try to practice them when you are late and find yourself stuck in a major traffic jam.

¤

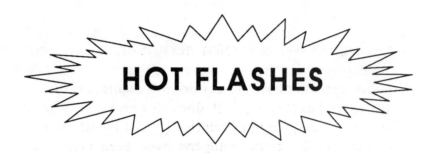

HOT FLASHES

➢ A strong thyroid-adrenal interdependence has been demonstrated time and again.
Febs Letters, 1991[18]

➢ Adrenal substances respond to emotional strain.
Journal of Neurochemistry, 1992[19]

➢ Stress causes abnormal enlargement of the adrenals and a detrimental change in the thymus.
Neuroscience and Behavioral Physiology, 1992[20]

➢ Emotional stress results in reactions in the hypothalamus and adrenals, among other problems.
Kardiologiia, 1992[21]

➢ Estrogens may be released from the adrenals and/or ovaries during psychological stress, contributing to excesses.
Neuroscience and Biobehavioral Reviews, 1992[22]

~~ ENDNOTES ~~ *The fantasy continues...*

The next segment of my fantasy doesn't require any yet-to-be-discovered technology. It does, however, require an extraordinary imagination. Picture, if you will, all the women for whom synthetic progestogens have been prescribed. Now they descend, en masse, on their doctors' doorsteps, demanding that their prescriptions be rewritten for *natural* progesterone. And—remember, this is fantasy—the doctors happily cooperate and rewrite all the prescriptions!

The crowds on the physicians' doorsteps and in their waiting rooms may increase as word spreads about the use of natural progesterone for conditions other than PMS, menopausal symptoms, and osteoporosis.

Or they may decrease, as people learn about self-help and even better—about *prevention.*

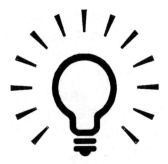

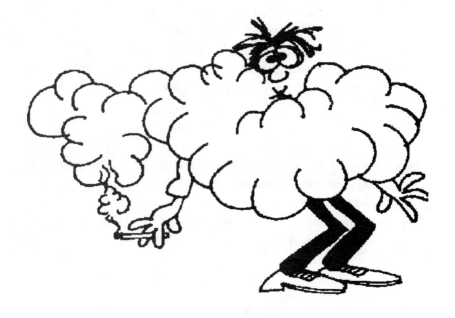

I wonder why I got that letter from the EPA warning me about my contribution to indoor pollution.

14

PROGESTERONE TREATMENT

PROGESTERONE FOR MENOPAUSE

If you were to tell me that you've done all the good things listed in the food and supplement chapters and have been for most of your life, I'd be very surprised if you had a problem with PMS, menopause, or osteoporosis. I'd also be very surprised if you were telling the truth! Let's be realistic—almost nobody in this society can follow such a strict regimen of prohibitions and special foods. So most of us need help. And that help may come in the form of plant-based natural progesterone.

The word progesterone was first proposed by William Allen and George Corner in 1934, when they isolated this newly discovered sex hormone. Since then, more than 5,000 plants have been identified as containing substances with progesterone-like chemistry. In 1943, Russel Marker successfully manufactured progesterone from the roots of Mexican yams. With minor conversion in the laboratory, the Mexican yam extract, *diosgenin*, has been made to match natural progesterone exactly. But the manufacture of cortisone and progestogens from the same raw materials attracted far more attention. The neglect of progesterone led Dr. Dalton to refer to it as "the forgotten hormone."[1]

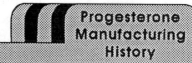

History of the Manufacture of Progesterone
(Outside the Human Body)

The principal source of the steroid chemical nucleus used in the drug industry is the plant kingdom. In the not too distant past, however, the source was from the gonads and adrenal glands of animals that were used as food by people. The amount of hormone present in these glands was extremely small. So large quantities of glands were required to isolate very minute quantities of the hormone. For example, one laboratory had to extract 625 kilograms of ovaries from 50,000 sows in order to obtain 20 milligrams of pure crystalline progesterone.

Today, the steroid industry represents the culmination of efforts by many scientists. Plant species rich in steroidal substances were discovered. Included is the Mexican yam. Using these *sapogenins*, the cost scaled down considerably. A vast amount of research resulted in improvement of the basic procedures over the years.

The recent success of several practitioners has helped us to catch up with this hormone. We are beginning to see the spotlight turned back in progesterone's direction.

When is the use of progesterone appropriate? *Like nearly all of us*, you may be among the women who could probably benefit from assistance, and progesterone could be the answer.

It's difficult not to be impressed with reports of improved well-being from the use of transdermal natural progesterone therapy. Less anxiety and depression, increased vitality and reduced sleep disturbances—not to mention enhanced sexual libido—are all benefits of a product with a track record of total safety![2]

Are you already on estrogen replacement therapy? Do you want to bail out? A slow weaning process is mandatory, preferably under a physician's care. If you are on Premarin, for example, you may be advised to cut down your intake by 10 to 15 percent each month simply by skipping days. (Alternating days may work better than dividing the tablets only because they are difficult to split.) As for patches, they can be worn for shorter periods of time, gradually diminishing the duration of their application.

If, however, you have made the decision to continue or to begin the traditional form of hormone or estrogen replacement therapy (HRT or ERT), it should be clear that natural progesterone used in conjunction with estrogen is called for. Most physicians now prescribe oral progestogens with the oral estrogen pill. Try to avoid synthetic progestogens— *ask your physician to recommend natural progesterone.* Although there is some uncertainty about absorbability with oral forms, it's possible to get good results with the right combination of diet, exercise, and balanced estrogen-progesterone therapy.

Robert Atkins, M.D., of New York City, prescribes estrogen for his menopause patients only if other treatments fail to reduce symptoms. And then he recommends just enough estrogen to reduce problems to a tolerable degree—not necessarily to eliminate them; he wants to keep the dose low. "Natural progesterone," he says, "is an absolute MUST to accompany estrogen therapy. Patients report desired changes in a week or two of the combined therapy." (Recovery takes longer with the use of natural progesterone alone, but avoids the possibility of side effects.) Dr. Atkins also recommends high doses of folic acid plus boron for anyone on estrogen replacement therapy.[3] (Again: high doses of folic acid should only be taken with a doctor's advisement.)

Another problem with synthetic progestogens involves glucose (blood sugar), metabolism. Natural progesterone is converted into corticosteroid hormones by your adrenal glands. These substances help to regulate your blood sugar metabolism. You may experience a drop in blood sugar if your progesterone is low. Low blood sugar causes the sensation of hunger, and you know how that feels—you're ready to jump on your child or mate for no reason. This scenario frequently occurs with the use of synthetic progestogens because the synthetics do *not* convert to corticosteroids. *To add insult to injury, they also lower your natural progesterone levels.*

Neils H. Lauersen, M.D., of New York's Mount Sinai Medical Center, advises that because synthetic progestogens may inhibit the concentration of natural progesterone, hormone imbalances are worsened. This is unfortunate, because these imbalances are no doubt "off" to begin with![4]

> Any standard medical text explains that estrogen's maximum benefit for osteoporosis is no more than a temporary reduction in the rate of osteoporotic bone resorption.

Physicians appear to be influenced, albeit inadvertently, by drug-company advertising rather than by information in their own textbooks. If you learn just a little about bone metabolism and about the functions of the osteoblasts and osteoclasts (as explained earlier), you can talk to your physician about bone loss. You might even tell your doctor that you know that natural progesterone stimulates osteoblasts and that you know that estrogen slightly restrains osteoclasts.

Chances are you now know as much about natural progesterone metabolism than most physicians. Don't hesitate to show these chapters to your doctor, pointing out the extensive medical journal citations and clinical validations included extensively throughout and at the back of this book.

When you intervene with estrogen you're adding a powerful hormone that has a direct effect on tissue all over your body. But progesterone is more of an intermediate building block. You're giving your endocrine system a tool to work with while leaving the natural control and regulation mechanisms in place. That explains why it's so much safer to use natural progesterone than estrogen. Remember our discussion of the huge dose of progesterone you made for yourself during pregnancy? Far from being harmful, it helped you feel great, even euphoric. And studies show that natural progesterone helps to prevent or reverse osteoporosis whether or not supplemental estrogen is also used.[5,6]

Recall that one traditional problem with the use of natural progesterone is the fact that your liver protects you from dietary hormones with first-pass removal during digestion. In her book *Once a Month,* Dr. Dalton lamented the lack of an easy way of getting progestogens into the bloodstream:

> *For many doctors progesterone is a forgotten hormone so far as treatment is concerned, and many doctors who use estrogen and know its possibilities and limitations are shy of using progesterone. One problem is that progesterone cannot be taken by mouth, as it is too quickly broken down in the liver, so it has to be given in other ways such as pessaries (tablets to be inserted into the vagina), suppositories (for use in the anus), injections, or implants. Recent work in India on monkeys has suggested that it is absorbed into the bloodstream when given by nasal administration. So who knows, we may yet be using it in aerosols or nasal sprays.*[7]

There is a way to circumvent the difficulty! Natural progesterone is dissolved in a moisturizing cream base that may also contain aloe vera, vitamin E, a humectifyer to preserve moisture, and even keratin (a principal constituent of epidermis, or skin) for connective tissues. Spreading the cream over a substantial area of skin is the method of application, so that the hormone can enter your blood *transdermally* (through your skin). The cream leaves no trace after a few minutes. Newer oil-based liquids also appear to sidestep the problem.

In *Cancer Causes and Control*, 1992, researchers advise that women currently using unopposed estrogen, estrogen and synthetic progestogens, or synthetic progestogens alone, are all at increased risk for breast cancer compared with never-users. According to this report, the addition of synthetic oral progesterone (more accurately, progestogen) does *not* remove the increased risk observed with current use of unopposed estrogen.[8] This is typical of an error in the use of the word *progesterone*, an inaccuracy made by many physicians. It cannot be overemphasized that side effects stem from *synthetic* progestogens and not from *natural* progesterone. The word *progesterone* refers only to the specific molecule as made by the ovary and should not be confused with the numerous synthetic substitutes.

As Dr. Lee explains:

> *There are no known side effects from natural progesterone which, as should be obvious to all, is the preferred form to use if supplementation is to be given.*
>
> *Estrogen does increase the risk of breast cancer over time and this risk can be reduced by progesterone, but not by all progestins. The various progestins differ in this regard. Both estrogen and most progestins increase intracellular sodium and water, leading to hypertension, whereas progesterone acts to prevent intracellular sodium and water, thus preventing hypertension and sparing the heart. Some progestins increase blood lipids, but natural progesterone does not. [Many physicians and researchers] confuse the synthetic progestins with natural progesterone.[9]*

Is it any wonder that breast cancer has increased so rapidly in recent years? Its victims in the United States alone could fill a 747 every day. And on every third day, the equivalent of a 747 full of women die from this avoidable disease.

Should you treat yourself with natural progesterone? Until recently, the short answer to this question was "No." At one time, the only way to get natural progesterone was to have it injected or to take it as a very inconvenient suppository or pessary. Oral forms were not natural.

The introduction of natural progesterone cream now provides a viable choice. Is it safe, then, to experiment with natural progesterone cream without medical supervision?

The clinical experiences of Dr. Lee and the other physicians I interviewed suggest an affirmative answer. Applying a small amount, totalling about an ounce of progesterone cream every month to the soft-skin areas of your body (such as breasts, neck, face, stomach, inside area of thighs, and upper inner arms) supplies a total of about 1,000 milligrams of natural progesterone. If a woman uses this quantity in two weeks, she waits until the next month to start the next ounce. Many patients are advised to apply the cream for the first ten days of every month. Others, concerned with infertility, apply the cream from Day 15 to Day 25 of their cycle. Dr. Lee suggests:

> Use a different part of your body each of four nights, then repeat. Once fat cells are saturated with progesterone, they won't accept any more, so vary the areas to which you apply the progesterone, allowing time for the progesterone to be absorbed into your bloodstream. The photon bone density test is a sure way to track your progress.

For hot flashes, the recommendation is one-fourth to one-half teaspoon of the cream at 15-minute intervals for one hour or until the flashes disappear. A severe case? Two drops of natural progesterone oil (in liquid form) should be held under the tongue one to two minutes at seven-to ten-minute intervals until the flashes stop.

Dr. Lee highly recommends its use even for women (like me) who live a prudent lifestyle and have never experienced menopausal symptoms. Dr. Lee reminds us that we are subject to stresses our bodies are not prepared for. We are using 3½-million-year-old genes in a late twentieth century world. He also reminds us that we cannot get enough natural progesterone or its precursors even if we eat the very best food available to us. Our diets cannot be good enough, regardless of heroic efforts.

When asked how long one should use the cream, Dr. Lee responds, "Until you are 96. Then we'll talk about it."

In addition to Mexican yams, diosgenin is also derived from soybean products (recall the lack of PMS and menopausal symptoms among Asians), and, occasionally from animal sources. In France, it is taken from human placenta.

PROGESTERONE FOR PMS

What about PMS? What if you've already tried everything, live the model lifestyle, eat the prudent diet—to the best of your ability—and still suffer every month? The damage done by half a lifetime of environmental assaults (not to mention your mother's lifestyle before and during her pregnancy) may be insurmountable if you use only the sometimes-blunt and slow-acting tools of natural or holistic methods described above. Besides, following the perfect lifestyle/diet may be impossible for perfectly good reasons. Don't feel guilty. Feel better! Natural progesterone could make the difference.

Varying degrees of PMS have been treated successfully with the use of natural progesterone cream by many physicians. Among them:

> ➤ Esther Kirk, M.D., in Westwood Village, California, notes that several PMS patients refer to progesterone cream as their "miracle cream."[10]

> ➤ Psychiatrist Louis Marx reports that, "In most cases the symptoms are eliminated. Certainly, I have not encountered any substance which is more effective than progesterone in relieving PMS."[11]

> ➤ Dr. Serafina Corsello says, "During the menstrual cycle my young women take one teaspoonful of progesterone cream from day 12 to day 28 and progesterone oil under the tongue in the event of pain or irritability. This treatment has made a tremendous difference. I personally wouldn't be without my progesterone cream."

➤ Dr. Richard Kunin says that some of his patients experience PMS relief in less than 15 minutes.[12] (He prescribes the progesterone in an oil-based form sublingually—under the tongue for quick absorption. Sublingual preparations MUST be absorbed just that way and should not be swallowed. Dr. Kunin feels that the stickiness of the oil-based natural progesterone is an advantage—it stays under the tongue until absorbed. One should, however, be certain that the supply is absolutely fresh. Oils, like the vitamin E used in some of these preparations, rancidify quickly. (Although vitamin E is an antioxidant, it can get rancid.)

➤ Dr. Lee says, "In my experience, natural progesterone is effective in the majority of cases of PMS, especially as part of a treatment program that includes proper diet and basic vitamin and mineral supplements. The beneficial change in the quality of life for these patients is remarkable."[13]

➤ Martin Milner, N.D., a naturopathic physician in Portland, Oregon, also uses an oil-based natural progesterone formula. His experience confirms his belief that the special oil suspension aids in proper absorption, but the taste is not exactly "cherry pie." Dr. Milner believes that it is imperative to check a woman's progesterone levels before and during administration so that adjustments in dosage can be made accordingly. He is astounded at the lack of testing done by physicians who prescribe estrogen with apparent abandon—especially when it's the progesterone that is more frequently deficient in pre-, peri-, and postmenopausal women.

For cramping at the onset of a period, several of these physicians advise the application of one-half teaspoon of the cream to the abdomen every 30 minutes until cramping subsides. If symptoms persist, they recommend adding the oil: two drops held under the tongue for 60 seconds at seven- to ten-minute intervals until symptoms are relieved. For PMS migraines, they suggest one-fourth to one-half teaspoon of the cream applied to the back of the neck and across the forehead and temples, plus two drops of the oil held under the tongue for 60 seconds at 15-minute intervals, if necessary. Transdermal application should be equally effective wherever the skin is smooth enough for the natural progesterone to be absorbed.

> Larger doses of natural progesterone are recommended to counter the PMS culprit: *high amounts of estrogen.*

How does natural progesterone work to relieve the burdensome symptoms of PMS? Turn back to Figure 6 on page 50, which shows the relative levels of estrogen and progesterone during a normal 28-day cycle, with Day 1 defined as the first day of menstruation. Notice the progesterone build-up after ovulation (normally at Day 14), which tapers off again before Day 1 of the next cycle. PMS generally occurs between ovulation and the beginning of menstruation, when serum levels of progesterone should be highest (days 14 to 28 on the chart).

> The average progesterone level after ovulation is lower in PMS sufferers than in those without symptoms.

What we *don't* know is exactly *why* progesterone deficiency occurs. It could be that your ovaries aren't performing their progesterone-producing function well enough. Or it could be a deficiency in one of the ovary-controlling hormones from your hypothalamus or pituitary gland controlling the ovaries. Or it may not be a progesterone deficiency at all, but a problem with too much estrogen compared with a normal amount of progesterone—in which case the addition of natural progesterone helps to normalize the ratio.

It may also be a simple and important reaction to stress. Without progesterone to thicken the uterine walls and to prepare them to receive a fertilized egg, a pregnancy is unlikely. As noted earlier, stress contributes to progesterone deficiency. It makes sense to me—would you really want to get pregnant during a period of high stress? I find this explanation attractively uncomplicated, but we don't really know if it's totally correct.

What we *do* know is that there is evidence that natural progesterone supplementation works to alleviate PMS in the majority of cases. We also know that synthetic progestogens, because they inhibit the concentration of natural progesterone, may heighten the imbalance of hormones and intensify PMS symptoms. A few of the progestogens in the marketplace are actually 2,000 times more potent than natural progesterone, which may be why some of them can make you feel worse than others.

Progesterone treatments have been accepted so completely in Great Britain that in three different murder trials, women have been "sentenced" to take progesterone. The defense? They committed violent crimes because they were premenstrual. Instead of going to jail, the women were remanded to their pharmacists.[14]

PROGESTERONE AND OTHER APPLICATIONS

Sex steroids, including progesterone, have effects on the anatomy and physiology of many nonreproductive organ systems. Here are some examples of the benefits of progesterone, apart from those demonstrated for PMS and menopause.

During Pregnancy

What about progesterone supplementation during pregnancy? There's some intriguing data about increased intelligence that sounds almost too exciting to be true. Here's an abstract of a paper that appeared in the *British Journal of Psychiatry* in 1976:

> *Children whose mothers received prenatal progesterone have been shown to be advanced in development at one year and to have greater academic achievement at nine to ten years. This study compares the educational attainments at 17 to 20 years of 34 progesterone children with 37 normal and 12 toxemic controls. More progesterone children continued schooling after 16 years compared with controls; higher proportion left school with...'A' level passes; the average number of passes per child was greater; and more obtained a university place. The best academic results were in those whose mothers had received over five grams of prenatal progesterone and for whom administration commenced before the sixteenth week and for whom treatment lasted longer than eight weeks.*

Objective measures of intelligence are necessarily very difficult to evaluate and are loaded with complicating factors. Yet this report is from a very credible source: a published paper by Dr. Dalton, the author of the landmark work that first identified PMS in 1953.[15]

Once again, the differences between natural progesterone and the synthetic progestogens must be addressed. If synthetic progestogen is harmful for an adult, there is no question about its harm for a small, growing fetus. But, as emphasized, natural progesterone functions very differently, and your body produces huge quantities during pregnancy.

As a contraceptive

Did you ever wonder why women who have had one ovary removed continue to ovulate every month? Didn't we assume that the ovaries take turns ovulating? Not exactly! After an egg is discharged, the progesterone build-up that occurs is responsible for sending a signal to the other ovary with a message that the egg-releasing is a *fait accomplis,* as indicated earlier. Progesterone is the messenger.

After ovulation, one of the results of the rapidly increasing progesterone level is to make both the mucous linings and vaginal fluid thick and sticky to a degree that prevents additional sperm from entering the womb. (If the ovulation has already resulted in fertilization, the fertilized egg will be up in the Fallopian tube near the ovary. The successful sperm will have entered the tube before the progesterone buildup begins.) So natural progesterone may also be effective as a contraceptive. I'm not suggesting that you rely on this method to prevent pregnancy, but be aware that progesterone supplementation before ovulation may have this effect.[16] If you want to become pregnant, and you are taking natural progesterone to alleviate PMS symptoms, administer your natural progesterone on days 14 to 26 of your cycle (after ovulation).

For Fertility

Although used for contraception, natural progesterone is able to trigger fertility in human spermatozoa, suggesting a clinical application in the treatment of the different techniques of assisted fertilization.[17] In other words, it helps to normalize out-of-order conception functions.

Natural progesterone supplementation can correct a luteal phase defect and result in an improved conception rate.[18] Note the suggestion above for its use during Days 14 to 26 following ovulation.

For Increased Sex Drive

I have already related the appealing story of the remote group of island people who consume large quantities of a tuber similar to the Mexican yam. The libido rate of these people is extraordinarily high, yet their population rate is surprisingly low. Perhaps this is the quintessential story that demonstrates both the love-making *and* the contraceptive propensities of natural progesterone. (To protect this island against a population explosion by foreigners, it will remain unidentified! For those who insist on following through, check the October 1992 issue of *National Geographic*.)[19]

Is there enough diosgenin in an American yam to be beneficial? If so, how many yams would you have to eat? Do you have enough of the nutrients necessary for your body to turn diosgenin into progesterone? To date, these issues haven't been explored.

> Because of nutrient-depleted soil and nutrient-depleting marketing delays (the time it takes to get food like Mexican yams from the garden to your table) my advice is to consider the transdermal cream.

For Asthma

Premenstrual asthma flare-up is a well known phenomenon which can be improved by progesterone.[20]

For Epilepsy

Dr. Dalton offers this encouraging information for epileptics: "One of the most satisfying experiences is to diagnose and treat a woman with premenstrual epilepsy. She can be treated with progesterone and freed from all anticonvulsant tablets with their many and unpleasant side effects."[21]

A more recent report in *Epilepsia*, published in 1991, confirms Dr. Dalton's conclusions: "Natural progesterone and other antiestrogenic agents constitute rational and effective adjuncts to epilepsy therapy.[22]

An even later study (*Epilepsy Research*, 1993) indicates that progesterone has an effect on epileptic seizure because of its barbiturate-like mechanism of action on brain metabolites.[23]

For Prostate Cancer

Why include information about prostate cancer in a book *for and about* women? With the increasing incidence of prostate problems, why not be informed? If your significant other isn't a male, what about your father, brother, cousin, or friend?

Here's the story: If a man has his testicles removed as a result of prostate cancer, or has an undescended testicle as a result of DES used by his mother during pregnancy, the loss of testosterone may lead to osteoporosis. This can be prevented or treated by natural progesterone replacement. Natural progesterone has no feminizing effects and will accomplish the same bone-building benefits as testosterone.[24]

For Endometrial Hyperplasia

Endometrial hyperplasia is the abnormal growth of cells in the mucous lining of the uterus. When women developed endometrial hyperplasia because of estrogen use they were observed to revert to normal endometrium when placed on natural progesterone.[25]

For Hypertension

As reported in the *Journal of Epidemiology*, 1990, research relating menopause and sex hormones to blood pressure conclude that progesterone is a protective factor for hypertension.[26] Synthetic progestogens and estrogens, however, have been associated with increased sodium content of body cells, leading to hypertension.[27]

For Skin Care

Dr. Atkins is especially enthusiastic about natural progesterone cream for skin care. He endorses its use because he finds it the best wrinkle-eradicator he's ever experienced.[28]

For Other Problems

Similar testimonials can be found regarding natural progesterone's effectiveness against polycystic breast disease (formation of many cysts) and cervical dysplasia (abnormal development of the cervix). These are potentially very serious conditions which require treatment plans directed by your physician.

¤

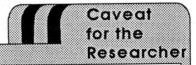

MEMOS

Caveat for the Researcher

Researcher Beware!

As my research on natural progesterone progressed, I could not help but be more and more impressed with its positive results—both clinically and in the laboratory. One exception surfaced, but after careful examination it was obvious that the conclusions of research that caught my attention left much to be desired. In this study, bone mineral response was checked *after* the participants spent a year on transdermal estradiol, and then again a year later after micronized progesterone was added orally (from Days 13 to 24).[29] (The process of micronizing reduces the progesterone to finer particles for easier absorption.)

Since the bone benefit observed was no different after the second year, it was determined that the progesterone had no effect. The graphs presented in the study, however, show that the mineral density of some bones tested *did actually increase*. Add to that a potential error percentage that exists with this form of testing, and then consider what might have happened if the researchers had used *transdermal* progesterone and/or if the participants were not given the estradiol. I myself could not conclude from this particular study that natural progesterone is ineffective for bone-building even though this was the end result cited. Physicians noting this study may be unaware of all the facts.

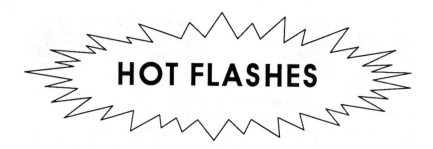

HOT FLASHES

➢ The transdermal route of hormone application may have fewer adverse liver effects.
Journal of Clinical Endocrinology and Metabolism,
1991.[30]

➢ Transdermal therapy represents an important advance in hormone therapy.
Drugs, 1990[31]

➢ The risk of cancer in long-term perimenopausal treatment with estrogen is not prevented by the addition of progestogens—especially after a few years.
New England Journal of Medicine, 1989[32]

➢ The risk of cancer with long-term perimenopausal estrogen treatment may be increased with the addition of progestogens.
New England Journal of Medicine, 1989[33]

➢ Natural progesterone helps to prevent the possible negative effects resulting from pituitary dysfunction.
Human Reproduction, 1992[34]

➤ Failure of current double-blind trials to relieve PMS with progesterone use is caused by
using low-dose synthetic progestogens.
Medical Hypotheses, 1990[35]

➤ Using natural progesterone as a contraceptive adds a new measure of safety for breast-
feeding mothers, since the amount of the steroid secreted in mother's milk is not effectively
absorbed by the infant.[36]
*Journal of Steroid Biochemistry and Molecular Bi-
ology, 1991*

➤ Women whose pregnancies end in miscarriages tend to have lower concentrations of
progesterone.
Fertility and Sterility, 1993[37]

➤ Progesterone supplementation may affect
pregnancy rates of in-vitro fertilization by increasing endometrial thickness, thereby en-
hancing receptivity for implantation.
Human Reproduction, 1992[38]

➤A 0.8-mg dose of the progestin ST 1435 administered transdermally once a day appears
to suppress ovulation.
Fertility and Sterility, 1992[39]

➤ Progesterone is essential for pregnancy.
Annals of Medicine, 1993[40]

➤ The normal monthly changes of female hormones can also affect the severity of responses to therapy in conditions such as asthma.
Journal of the American Medical Womens Association, 1993[41]

➤ The advantages of delivering drugs through the skin for systemic therapy have been widely recognized and represent a growing sector in drug development.
Annals of Medicine, 1993[42]

➤ Transdermal delivery of steroids is a rapidly expanding field. In various clinical situations where hormonal replacement therapy is needed, this route of administration is a real breakthrough—especially considering the relative toxicity of some steroids when given orally.
Annals of Medicine, 1993[43]

➤ Progesterone has been demonstrated to be a good candidate for transdermal delivery.
Annals of Medicine, 1993[44]

➤ Most of the harmful adverse effects of ERT have been related to the absence of progestational balance.
Drugs, 1990[45]

➤ During the past decade, several isolated reports have linked an increased incidence of breast cancer with the use of synthetic progestins.
Cancer, 1993[46]

~~ ENDNOTES ~~ *The fantasy continues...*

Even in our fantasy, it's not easy to disentangle the complexities of menstrual, menopausal, and aging disorders, now so commonplace in our society. All long-term consequences of growing older are more amenable to prevention than to cure. That, of course, is easier said than done.

Dr. Lee's summary statements on estrogen and natural progesterone plus the concluding comments in the next segment may help you make your decision. Dr. Lee's Summary Statements:

> *Estrogen stimulates the breast, creates proliferative endometrium, causes salt and fluid retention, increases body fat, interferes with thyroid hormone, causes depression and headaches, increases blood clotting, diminishes libido, impairs blood-sugar control, causes decline of zinc and retention of copper, reduces oxygen levels in all cells, causes endometrial cancer, increases the risk of breast cancer, and slightly restrains osteoclasts.*

> *Natural progesterone protects against fibrocysts, maintains secretory endometrium, functions as a natural diuretic, helps use fat for energy, stimulates thyroid hormone action, is a natural antidepressant, normalizes blood clotting, restores libido, normalizes blood sugar levels, normalizes zinc and copper levels, restores proper cell oxygen levels, prevents endometrial cancer, helps prevent breast cancer, stimulates osteoblasts, is necessary for the survival of the embryo, and is a precursor of cortisone synthesis.*

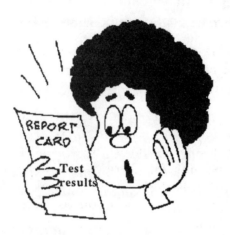

"Tony, you failed your health test.
The four food groups are NOT
McDonald's, Kentucky Fried Chicken,
Dunkin' Doughnuts, and Pizza Hut!"

15

CHOICES

With all the information cited in these pages as background, we come full circle to the title of this book: *Hormone Replacement Therapy—Yes or No?* Let's review some of the facts.

It's a tough decision because in spite of all the proved disadvantages, the medical literature indicates that estrogen-progestogen hormone replacement therapy has been confirmed as an effective prevention for osteoporosis in postmenopausal women. But you are better informed now. It's still a tough decision, because hormone therapy involves judgment in weighing the pros and cons.

No one dies from vaginal atrophy, bladder dysfunction, or hot flashes. Quality of life and marriage, however, could be improved by relieving these symptomatic conditions with some form of hormone therapy.[1] Cancer, of course, is life-threatening.

After surveying current literature on hormone therapy in postmenopausal women, the medical journal *Family Practice* came to this less-than-satisfying conclusion: *Hormone therapies in postmenopausal women are controversial and provoke more questions than answers.*

In 1991, the Nurses' Health Study revealed a 46 percent increase in ischemic stroke risk among nurses using estrogen replacement therapy, despite the fact that this group was comprised of women with less diabetes, less cigarette smoking, and less adiposity than those not using estrogen.[2]

Estrogens can slow the process of bone loss, but is the increased risk of breast cancer sufficient to preclude their use? A combination of estrogen and synthetic progestogens may, according to some of the literature, avoid the increased risk of uterine cancer. But what are the effects of *long-term* administration? Do the potential benefits of hormone therapy justify the costs and treatment of large numbers of women who, without therapy, may never have developed complications attributable to lack of estrogen? Given these uncertainties, is postmenopausal administration of hormones reasonable or wise? The current literature does not provide adequate answers to these questions mainly because it generally does not consider *natural* progesterone as part of the protocol.[3]

Are physicians paying enough attention to the contraindications of HRT? According to generally accepted research, traditional hormone replacement therapy should not be used for women who have had:

> ➤ breast cancer
> ➤ thrombophlebitis
> ➤ hypertension
> ➤ gallstones
> ➤ diabetes
> ➤ undiagnosed abnormal genital bleeding.[4]

There's more! If you or close members of your family are cancer-prone, you may be apprehensive about the relationship of postmenopausal use of estrogen and endometrial cancer. Keep in mind that rates of endometrial cancer have risen sharply. Fluid retention, breast enlargement, and growth of preexisting uterine tumors have been noted. If these are familiar problems for you or close family members, estrogen therapy is contraindicated.

Breast tissue ages according to hormonal (primarily estrogen) exposure. Because of this fact and other similar variations studied internationally, *the incidence rates of breast cancer can actually be predicted throughout the world.*[5] Although association is not proof of cause, researchers are taking a hard look at these parallel statistics.

Estrogen therapy requires annual tests for blood evaluation. Urine and breasts need to be examined on a regular basis. Your physician is aware of the possibility of stimulating blood in urine, necessitating frequent checks. Women on long-term estrogen therapy appear to have about a 30-percent greater chance of developing breast cancer. Periodic endometrial biopsies for early detection of pre-malignant or malignant endometrial changes may be recommended.[6]

In making your decision, recall that estrogens do not restore lost bone and that withdrawal of estrogen therapy is followed by significant bone loss—thus suggesting that therapy must be ongoing for many years.[7] You become a patient—not only as long as you continue therapy, but also after you stop therapy. Even more depressing, the positive estrogen effects do not last more than three to five years.

As noted, several of the nutrition-oriented physicians I interviewed indicated that they prescribe very small amounts of estrogen only if hot flashes and vaginal dryness are unbearable. They also prescribe it for the rare osteoporotic patient for whom natural progesterone alone may not be sufficiently effective. These physicians are so concerned about estrogen therapy, they prescribe doses only to the point of making symptoms tolerable—but not necessarily to eliminate the discomfort totally. Low-dose transdermal forms of estrogen therapy may avoid some of the complications of higher-dose oral therapy.[8]

CYCLIC ESTROGEN: ADDING PROGESTOGENS

Your physician may be influenced by tempting reports about reduced risks of estrogen therapy when progestogens are added.[9] *Cyclic* estrogen administration prior to menopause is an effort to imitate nature. The patient uses progesterone for ten days to initiate endometrial sloughing and then stops but continues to use estrogen the entire month.

With this therapy, a woman may menstruate into her sixties and seventies. The disadvantage is the monthly withdrawal bleeding, and this would surely be considered a very serious side effect were it not for the fact that you've had your entire adult life to get used to it. Whether or not this does actually reduce the risk of cancer is still debatable. But the handwriting is on the wall and it doesn't bode well.

The results of a well-designed study to assess the side effects of medroxyprogesterone in replacement therapy, published in *Obstetrics and Gynecology*, warns: *Cyclic progestogen therapy appears to have preceded detailed evaluation of possible adverse side effects of progestogens.*[10] A warning that perhaps we have "jumped in" too soon!

When statements are made indicating that the combined therapy reduces risk, it is not clear whether the reduction is *to the level of* or *below* the risk observed in an untreated population. All progestogens may cause physical, psychological, and metabolic side effects. In fact, side effects are common and there is a high incidence of bleeding in the first few months, which is unacceptable to many patients. (Once again—a reminder that progestogens are synthetic, and differ from natural progesterone.)

The March 1993 issue of the *FDA Consumer* discusses Depo-Provera, the quarterly contraceptive. Depo-Provera inhibits the production of another hormone, gonadotropin, which in turn, prevents ovulation. Depo-Provera also causes changes in the lining of the uterus that make pregnancy less likely. Note the following statements in this FDA-published journal:

➤ A link between Depo-Provera and breast cancer was first considered in the early 1970s in test animals. The studies were regarded as not applicable to humans. (Why not? The results of endless other similar studies are!)

➤ According to testimony presented to the *Fertility and Maternal Health Drugs Advisory Committee* of the FDA, June 1992, trials demonstrating safety of the product were conducted in countries with breast cancer rates less than half that of the United States and therefore can't be accurately applied to women in this country.[11]

➤ Only three epidemiologic studies were done on Depo-Provera and breast cancer, and all three raised a red flag.[12]

➤ The bone density in 30 women who had been using Depo-Provera for at least five years was *less* than the bone density of other women of similar age.[13]

The FDA report noted that a professor with the Department of Obstetrics and Gynecology at the University of Southern California School of Medicine, said, "Oh, these women must have had preexisting tumors." (Arggghhhhh!!!) The National Women's Health Network disagrees with the benign conclusions of the researchers promoting Depo-Provera as safe.[14] What is Depo-Provera? *Synthetic progestogen!*

Even though several risks such as endometrial and breast cancer associated with continuous ERT are reported to be significantly reduced with the use of cyclic progestogens, it hasn't been used long enough for conclusive evidence.[15] How do *you* feel about being a guinea pig?

SEQUENTIAL OR CONTINUOUS?

If you do decide on the prescribed replacement combination of estrogen plus synthetic progestogen, the next question is: Should it be continuous or sequential? Some postmenopausal women receiving sequential treatment develop PMS-like symptoms when synthetic progestogen is added.[16] Continuous combined estrogen and progestogen preparations eliminate the inconvenience of regular progestogen-induced withdrawal bleeding.[17] Any breakthrough bleeding occurring after a period of prolonged amenorrhea must be investigated by means of endometrial biopsy.[18] This makes you more than a participant—*you must become a patient.*

The continuous protocol has been eagerly embraced by women who don't want to be encumbered with the need to remember what day it is and when to take what. Many physicians, favoring compliancy, recommend what is easiest—*not necessarily what is good for your body.*

THE CHOICE

So when your doctor advocates estrogen treatment, you have a serious choice to make. You can agree to follow the advice, recognizing that when your hormones are being manipulated, you are handing over responsibility, which may be exactly what you want to do. Being the passive recipient of your doctor's choice of treatment may work for you. Not everyone wants to be in charge or make the changes.

Or, you may want to exert more control over your life. Do you want to make choices? Are you able to make beneficial changes in terms of both your behavior and the effects of your mind on your body? Honest answers to these questions will help you to make the right personal decision. It's not a matter of right or wrong. What you feel is best for *you* is the important factor.

If you settle on a supplement-and-exercise regimen on your own, you make *yourself* accountable, in which case you may have to be much more earnest about lifestyle changes. It may take awhile before you are relieved of uncomfortable symptoms—unless you have been lucky enough to have been eating *real* food, have been taking the *right* kind of supplements, and engaging in *correct* exercise before the onset of menopause.

Have you considered yourself the victim of bad luck or bad genes? Or do you think you are among those whose genes are good enough to circumvent the hazards of our current environment? If you identify with the former you should know that one *can* intercept heredity. Those in the latter category comprise less than two percent of the world's population.

If you are suffering from excessive sweating and flushes, it may not be an easy choice. One of the benefits of estrogen is a quick relief of hot flashes. Estrogen can make a big difference in your sleep; because of the reduction in flashes, there are fewer awakenings during the night. When you are exhausted from lack of sleep, the benefit of a restful night can be a powerful influence.

Not only is symptomatic relief (reduced frequency of sweating episodes, sleep disturbance and hot flushes), observed during treatment, but there are also improvements in terms of energy and emotions. Improvement in well-being, anxiety, depression, vitality, health and self-control takes place, and women experience less tension and more satisfaction.[19,20]

Can these advantages be achieved another way, thereby eliminating the side effects of the usual HRT? I know they can.

The use of postmenopausal hormones has been associated with a reduced risk of death from cardiovascular disease. *But the same protective effect provided by postmenopausal hormone therapy has been seen in women who experience natural menopause* (that is, menopause without the use of hormone therapy). This was the conclusion after research on the reduction of cardiovascular disease-related mortality among postmenopausal women who use hormones, reported in the *American Journal of Obstetrics and Gynecology*, 1991.[21]

I remind you again that the risks associated with estrogen therapy are clearly related to length of use. There is an apparent latent period of three to six years, after which the chances of incurring problems increase rapidly.

> Regardless of your decision, there are positive steps you can take to mitigate the potential dangers of estrogen therapy or the hazards of increased fractures, already outlined in previous pages.

Several aware practitioners note that side effects are reduced, if not eliminated, with the use of *natural* progesterone rather than the synthetic variety so commonplace today. They and their patients acclaim natural progesterone. Most physicians, however, are not getting this message. A brand-new indictment and analysis of medical practices, written by a physician (M. Konner, *Medicine at Crossroads*), still refers to progesterone as the *pregnancy hormone*.[22]

CHINESE MEDICINE AND HERBOLOGY

In this era of interest in Eastern medicine and the use of herbs, I would be remiss not to mention Chinese medicine and herbology. Dr. Herb Kandel, a licensed acupuncturist and Doctor of Oriental Medicine who practices in Santa Maria, California, contributed the following information:

"Herbs can improve general health as well as reduce common menopausal symptoms. Generally speaking, herbs are gentle on the body for two reasons: they are absorbed more slowly than single chemical extracts or synthetic pharmaceutical drugs; and constituents in herbs have multiple ingredients which are often counterbalancing to the active ingredients in that herb. The complex nature of herbal medicines may also explain certain herbs' ability to have self-regulating effects on the body. For example, the Chinese herb Dang Gui (Angelica sinensis) has properties which can both constrict an overly relaxed uterus and soften a cramping uterus. This ability of certain herbs to have multiple properties, and thus help the body self-regulate is evern more prominent in well-formulated herbal combinations.

"All herbs are not necessarily benignly good for you just because they are natural. Some herbs have very strong effects and should only be taken with professional guidance and for a limited period of time. Other herbs, with mild effects, can be taken regularly as a beverage tea or as supplements.

"There are three factors which can help you to choose herbs wisely: 1) an understanding of the qualities, actions, and common uses of each herb; 2) any potential adverse effects of each herb; and 3) knowledge of your own body's strengths, weaknesses and particular needs. Here is some information on herbs that have proved to be useful during menopause and for PMS.

"Chaste Berries or Vitex (Agnus castus). Vitex is the single most important western herb for regulating the period and reducing menopausal distress. Vitex stimulates the pituitary and helps the body produce progesterone. This herb has a balancing effect on estrogens while favoring progesterone. It is useful before menopause to normalize periods for as long as possible, as well as to treat painful periods. It is also effective in treating various problems associated with menopause.

"Dang Gui (Angelica sinensis). Dang Gui is a primary herb in Chinese medicine for treating menstrual irregularities, including delayed menses, pain during menstruation, and fatigue due to blood loss or deficiency. It has been adopted more widely in the west to treat menopausal syndromes but should not be used if excessive bleeding is present. Research shows that this herb has a normalizing effect on the muscles of the uterus, increases the metabolism of the liver, reduces atherosclerosis in arteries (animal studies) and has proved effective for various pain syndromes. Studies do not demonstrate an estrogenic effect as has been reported by some. In fact, clinical evidence points to progesterone production, since women who take this herb alone in a dose too high often report midcycle bleeding and light-headedness or grogginess. It is best taken in a formula or with professional guidance. Dang Gui can also be added to soups. Please note that the western relative of Dang Gui, Angelica archangelica, often called *angelica,* has fewer anti-spasmodic properties. It is not generally indicated for menopause and is contra-indicated during pregnancy.

"Black Cohosh (Cimicifuga racemosa). Black cohosh is very high in potassium and has a vasodilatory effect. Its effects include those of anti-inflammation and gentle sedation. Useful for menstrual pains and for reducing hot flashes, this herb lowers blood pressure and relaxes the muscles, as

shown in animal studies. In Chinese medicine, it is used for swelling in the mouth, such as canker sores and swollen or painful gums, and for the early stage of measles. Some physicians warn that Black Cohosh is specifically estrogenic, and therefore, unopposed with progesterone, risks endometrial buildup. Studies have not been done to demonstrate that it can cause endometrial cancer. Overdose can cause headaches, dizziness, and tremors (and pathogenic erections in males). If taken for a prolonged period of time, it should be used in a well-rounded formula with other herbs. Note: Blue Cohosh (Caulophyllum thalictroides) has similar properties but is less estrogenic and more pain-relieving in nature, and is a safer option if used individually.

"Siberian Ginseng (Eleutherococcus senticosus). This herb is a member of the ginseng family, with distinctively different effects from panax ginseng. Siberian ginseng is useful for increasing energy level and promoting enhanced tolerance to stress [as described more fully in Betty Kamen's booklet, *Siberian Ginseng: Up-to-Date Research on the Fabled Tonic Herb*]. It is useful for menopausal women who suffer from chronic fatigue or illness, frequent colds or flus, and sensitivity to emotional and environmental stress. Siberian ginseng must be taken on an ongoing basis for several weeks to notice the effects. Most women report feeling more resilient at an appropriate dose, or restless with increased irritability if the dose is too high. Here is one herb that can be safely taken as an individual herb. Product concentrations vary; start with the lowest recommended dose and adjust the dose according to how you feel. Note: Panax Ginseng should be avoided for most women during menopause, as should Korean ginseng, which can elevate blood pressure and may increase endometrial build up. [So if you've read literature indicating that women shouldn't take ginseng, keep all of these facts in mind, especially concerning the advantages of Siberian ginseng.]

"Herbs for Nervous Tension and Insomnia. Catnip, chamomile, passion flower, lemon balm, and hops are all gentle herbs which can be used to promote calmness and improve sleep. These herbs can be steeped in tea (low dose) on a regular basis over a long period of time. They are widely available as tea blends or as loose tea in health food stores. Valerian root has stronger sedative properties and can be used temporarily for particularly stressful times, but should not be used consistently over a long period. Valerian and skullcap can be useful in the process of withdrawal from drugs or alcohol.

"Advice for all herbal sedatives: avoid habituation, use sedatives in combination for more effectiveness, use herbs to reinforce natural cycles of rest (after work, before bed), and avoid use during pregnancy.

"As for Chinese medicine, it is best to consult a trained practitioner when choosing to use Chinese herbal formulas for menopausal symptoms. The following, however, are Chinese herbs which can be safely added to soups or stews.

"Cooked Rehmannia (Rehmanniae glutinosae). Traditional indications: replenishes blood and essence; relieves weakness, fatigue, dryness, anemia, irregular uterine bleeding, dizziness; strengthens bones and marrow; moistens tissues. This herb is rich in oils which contain essential fatty acids. Note: Because of its stickiness, it is often combined with specific herbs to aid digestion and has a mild, sweet, earthy flavor.

"Cornus (Cornus officinalis). Traditioanl indications: stabilizes 'kidney essence'; checks excessive sweating; strengthens bones and tendons; relieves frequent urination, dizziness, and excessive menstrual flow; enhances libido and fertility; stengthens low back and knee weakness.

"*Peony (Paeoniae lactiflorae)*. Traditional indications: nourishes the blood and calms the liver; indicated for menstrual dysfuntion, uterine bleeding, pain, especially spasms, cramps, or abdominal pains, night sweats, edginess, irritability, and mood swings.

"So you see that herbal and Chinese medicines can be useful in helping women journey through menopause in a more comfortable and self-empowered manner."

Herb Kandel,
Santa Maria, California

We are grateful to Dr. Kandel for his vast experience and insights, and, especially, for his generous contribution to this book.

TWO IMPORTANT QUESTIONS ANSWERED

What if you've had a hysterectomy?
If your uterus has been removed, but your ovaries have been left intact, you should be aware that within two to three years after such an operation, ovaries stop producing hormones. Adding natural progesterone cream and taking other measures to insure healthy and functioning adrenal glands is mandatory. If your ovaries have been removed, natural progesterone cream can be as beneficial as for women experiencing PMS or menopausal symptoms.

What if you're on birth control pills containing synthetic progesterone?
It is not a good idea to mix progesterones.

¤

THE WANING EFFECT OF POSTMENOPAUSAL ESTROGEN THERAPY ON OSTEOPOROSIS

As we go to press for the second edition of this book, the October 14, 1993 issue of the *New England Journal of Medicine* published, as its lead article, the results of research demonstrating the waning effect of postmenopausal estrogen therapy on osteoporosis. The article reminds us that almost all physicians and their patients believe that estrogen treatment can prevent osteoporosis. What we now know, however, is that in women more than 75 years old, there is little difference in bone density between women who had taken estrogen and those who had not. The research also validates that most osteoporotic fractures occur at an advanced age. The average age at hip fracture among postmenopausal women is 80 years!

Given these results, the researchers conclude that estrogen therapy in the first decade after menopause cannot be expected to protect against osteoporotic fractures many years later. They also validate, once again, what has been stated in earlier chapters here: the reduction in the risk of hip fracture associated with estrogen treatment dissipates after treatment is stopped. Once again, *estrogen treatment for 5 to 10 years soon after menopause is unlikely to preserve bone density or to prevent fractures in old age.*

The researchers suggest an alternative to the current trend of "estrogen-izing" all women: "Start estrogen after osteoporotic fracture, an effective strategy that targets easily identified women who have a high risk of recurrent fracture and are likely to comply with treatment...Another alternative is to start estrogen treatment many years after menopause...Other effects of estrogen treatment should be considered...including a possible increase in the risk of breast cancer." Not exactly my recommendations, but certainly a step forward!

MEMOS

What doctors read

One way to get a glimpse of what the doctors are thinking is to look at what they are reading. Despite the controversy, side effects, and lack of full understanding, the following messages appeared in recent issues of prestigious medical journals. This is what your doctors write and read. What do you think?

➤"Replacement therapy is the *assignment* of the gynecologist in order to protect the skeletal system."[23]

➤"An enhanced tendency to exhaustion in menopause is dependent on *psychosocial* factors that correspond to a typically 'feminine' role enactment as postulated by social convention."[24]

➤"Menopause is a medical condition; *natural approaches to menopause are less preferable;* women should take ERT for hot flashes. A systematic educational approach could influence women's willingness to take ERT."[25]

➤"*All* women should be followed by a gynecologist."

(The emphasis above is mine.) The practice of treating women as they go through one of life's most natural phases is now referred to as the emerging field of *menopause medicine.*

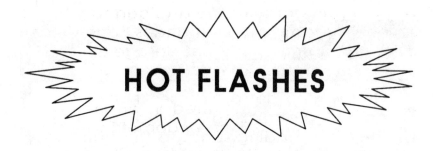

HOT FLASHES

➤ Estrogen and progesterone therapy may protect bones because they decrease magnesium excretion significantly. The effect is related to estrogen dose.

Magnesium and Trace Elements, 1991-92[26]

➤ Prenatal exposure to androgen-based synthetic progestogen exerts a masculinizing and/or defeminizing influence on human behavioral development.

Psychoneuroendocrinology, 1991[27]

➤ Major compliance problems of replacement therapy are alleged weight gain, resumption of withdrawal bleeding, and developing breast or endometrial cancer.

International Journal of Clinical Pharmacology, Therapy, and Toxicology, 1992[28]

➤ Cessation of estrogen therapy restores bone loss.

American Journal of Obstetrics and Gynecology, 1992[29]

➤ The addition of a progestogen may result in the return of menses, reducing compliance among the older female population.

American Journal of Obstetrics and Gynecology, 1992[30]

➤ Among the drawbacks ascribed to ERT are serious metabolic disturbances, particularly after oral administration of estrogens.

Annals of Medicine, 1993[31]

➤ Estrogens are implicated in an increased incidence of breast and endometrial cancer. Synthetic progestins can cause some estrogen-like effects (such as bone preservation), but studies show that some formulations place some groups of women at greater risk of having breast cancer.

Cancer, 1993[32]

➤ The long-term effect of postmenopausal estrogen therapy on bone density is not known.

New England Journal of Medicine, 1993[33]

➤ Estrogen therapy may become increasingly irrelevant as women approach the age at which the risk of fracture is highest.

New England Journal of Medicine, 1993[34]

➤ There are estrogen-dependent and age-dependent components of bone loss. By the age of 70, the age-dependent component predominates.

Journal of Clinical Endocrinology & Metabolism, 1990[35]

➤ Five or even 10 years of early postmenopausal estrogen therapy would have a trivial residual effect on bone mineral density at age 75.

Bone Mineral, 1990[36]

~~ ENDNOTES ~~ *From fantasy to reality!*

Twenty-three percent of hospitalization is iatrogenic—caused by a doctor. It is no wonder that a survey published in *New England Journal of Medicine* indicates that *unconventional medical help is sought by one-third of the United States population.* Americans made 425 million visits to such providers in 1990—compared with 388 million visits to all family doctors, internists, and other primary care physicians combined.

According to the report, patients rarely tell their physicians of their extracurricular unorthodox medical ventures. Three-quarters of the money spent is out of their own pockets and is not reimbursed by insurance companies. Unorthodox therapies are those that are not often taught at medical schools or practiced in hospitals. The people most likely to use such therapy are well-educated, middle-income folk.

Dr. Joe Jacobs, the new director of the National Institute of Health's Office of Alternative Medicine, said the popularity of alternative medicine demonstrates a hunger among Americans for more humane and less invasive treatments than those ordinarily practiced by standard doctors. Jacobs was most disturbed by the finding that 72 percent of those using unconventional therapies did not bother telling their doctors. "Some of these alternative therapies take a holistic and more caring view of a patient," he said.[37]

The question remains: Should you treat yourself with natural progesterone?

I'm lucky. I don't have to answer the question of whether or not to apply natural progesterone cream for myself because I have access to a number of physicians who think the way I do about nutrition, lifestyle, and health. In other words, not only do I go to a doctor I can trust, but my physician cooperates with me and even advocates many of the new and sometimes unconventional approaches that I believe are best. So my choice is easy.

But what if your doctor is less agreeable? What if your doctor is more conservative, is not aware of the latest findings in this area, doesn't respond well to suggestions from a patient, or is antagonistic to the use of natural progesterone or any other treatment you may decide to use?

It would be easy for me to simply say, "Find another doctor." This is not practical advice for many. You may not have *any* physician whom you see regularly, let alone easy access to an *acceptable* one. Finding a specialist who will work with you on a treatment regimen considered unorthodox may be out of the question.

Ultimately, we all have to be our own doctors. What we eat and how we live contributes far more to our long-term health than anything a medical doctor will ever be able to do for us. Of course there are obvious exceptions, where major interventions are life-saving. I think you get the point. The responsibility for good health is primarily your own. Hopefully, you'll act *before* you begin to notice the first faint rumblings of trouble.

Specific advice? Know your body as well as you possibly can, and do what *you* believe is best. Even if your physician is downright hostile to the use of natural progesterone or any other treatment you may decide to use, don't cut off communications. Keep your doctor informed of your personal health decisions and their results, if you possibly can. The flow of information will help to give us all the knowledge to stay healthy.

Dear Dr. Lee,

Thank you so much for suggesting the use of natural progesterone cream. I am feeling so much better — no more hot flashes, no more sleepless nights.

My daughter thanks you, too. The cream has solved her PMS problems.

Sincerely,
Jane Smith

P.S. Oh, and as for libido, again, my thanks (and my husband thanks you, too!).

HOW TO USE THE FOOD TABLES

The food tables that follow list the calcium and phosphorous content of 157 common foods and food products, the silicon content of 73 fruits and vegetables, and the boron content for 5 representative vegetables.

You can use the calcium/phosphorous table to insure that your diet is providing enough calcium, and especially to monitor the amount of phosphorous in comparison to the amount of calcium. Keep in mind that a natural diet—the diet that our bodies are designed to thrive on—contains only a little bit more phosphorous than calcium. Too much phosphorous in comparison to calcium interferes with incorporating new calcium into bone structure. Even if your bones are old, you need this supply of new calcium to make up for the calcium that is constantly being removed for use by other tissues.

The first calcium and phosphorus columns in the table are under the label "mg per 100 grams." There are 28 grams in an ounce, so 100 grams is about four ounces, or roughly a portion the size of your fist. A milligram is one one-thousandth of a gram. So if we had pure calcium, the table would indicate 100,000 milligrams per 100 grams. 100 milligrams per 100 grams, a more typical value for vegetables, means that the calcium content of the food is one part in one thousand, or one-tenth of a percent, by weight. Alfalfa sprouts, topping the list at 1,754 milligrams of calcium per 100 grams of food, is 17.5 parts per thousand, or 1.75 percent calcium by weight.

The calcium and phosphorous columns on the right side of the table, under the label "mg per serving," might be more useful for menu planning. Here the amounts are corrected by the typical serving size, as indicated in the far right column.

You should include at least 1,000 milligrams of calcium in your diet every day. Don't be tempted to concentrate on the dairy products, though. For reasons that are not fully understood, absorption and assimilation of calcium from dairy sources are not as good as from grain and vegetable sources.

The "bad" and "good" columns of the table are useful for assessing the amount of phosphorous as compared to calcium. Foods with more calcium and less phosphorous have a higher number under the "good" label. This number is simply the ratio of calcium-to-phosphorous. (The label on top of the column uses the chemical symbols P and Ca for phosphorous and calcium.) A higher number under "Ca/P" is a better food for helping your body maintain the proper calcium-to-phosphorous ratio. The "bad" column is the inverse ratio, phosphorus-to-calcium. A high number here works against you.

Take some time to study the tables. Note that many foods you may have associated with good nutrition have high numbers in the "bad" column. Garlic, for example, scores 7.0 bad points, and mushrooms are 11.3! It would be a mistake to avoid these foods because of this ratio (garlic, in particular, is a food I consider essential to good health). On this scale, fish doesn't look too good, either, but fish should remain a major component of your diet (broiled or baked, not fried, please).

So use the table to find good foods that will supply you with needed calcium without increasing the phosphorus burden. Note the stand-out foods in the "good" column, like cranberries, olives, and oranges. Kelp is an extremely valuable seasoning, and can also assist in reducing sodium intake. Alfalfa is an unbeatable source of calcium without much phosphorous, and a number of other vegetables like collard leaves and Swiss chard have excellent Ca/P ratios.

The tables for silicon show the amount of this element, in mg per 100 grams, for various fruits. No guideline is available for recommended daily intake, but it makes sense to give the foods that are high in silicon a special place on your shopping list. Dare I suggest "an apple a day...?"

Data for boron is hard to find, probably because the boron content of foods varies tremendously with the boron content of the soil in which it is grown. The tables show high and low values after testing several different samples of each food. It's probably safe to say that the consequences of modern agriculture techniques include less boron in our foods than the more traditional methods of farming. This is a negative health factor. Here is one of the best arguments for buying organic produce from small farms. There is still no guarantee that the boron content will be sufficient, but at least by diversifying the sources of your food you can improve the odds.

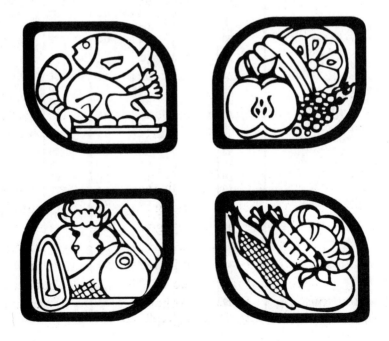

VEGETABLES	mg per 100 grams		P/Ca	Ca/P	mg per serving		serving
	calcium	phosph.	(bad)	(good)	calcium	phosph.	size
alfalfa	1754	251	0.1	7.0	1989	284	4 oz.
artichoke, cooked	51	69	1.4	0.7	58	78	4 oz.
asparagus, cooked	21	50	2.4	0.4	6	14	1 oz.
asparagus, uncooked	22	63	2.9	0.4	6	18	1 oz.
baked potatoes, with skin	9	65	7.2	0.1	20	147	8 oz.
beets, boiled	14	23	1.7	0.6	16	26	4 oz.
broccoli, cooked	88	62	0.7	1.4	100	70	4 oz.
Brussles sprouts, cooked	32	72	2.2	0.4	37	82	4 oz.
cabbage, cooked	130	230	1.8	0.6	147	261	4 oz.
carrots, raw	37	36	1.0	1.0	42	41	4 oz.
cauliflower, raw	25	56	2.2	0.4	28	64	4 oz.
celery, raw	39	28	0.7	1.4	44	32	4 oz.
chard	81	36	0.4	2.3	92	41	4 oz.
collard leaves & stems	203	82	0.4	2.5	230	93	4 oz.
corn, canned or cooked	4	48	12.0	0.1	5	54	4 oz.
cucumber, raw, unpeeled	26	28	1.1	0.9	29	32	4 oz.
dandelion greens	375	148	0.4	2.5	106	42	1 oz.
eggplant, steamed	11	26	2.4	0.4	13	30	4 oz.
French fried potatoes	15	111	7.4	0.1	34	251	8 oz.
garlic	29	202	7.0	0.1	8	57	1 oz.
green beens, cooked	50	37	0.7	1.3	57	42	4 oz.
green lima beens, raw	52	142	2.7	0.4	59	161	4 oz.
green peas, canned	20	66	3.3	0.3	23	75	4 oz.
green peas, fresh cooked	23	99	4.3	0.2	26	112	4 oz.
green peas, frozen	19	86	4.5	0.2	22	98	4 oz.
kale leaves	249	73	0.3	3.4	282	83	4 oz.
kidney beans	46	91	2.0	0.5	53	103	4 oz.
lettuce, iceberg	20	22	1.1	0.9	23	25	4 oz.
mung bean sprouts, raw	20	64	3.2	0.3	23	73	4 oz.
mushrooms, cooked or canned	6	68	11.3	0.1	7	77	4 oz.
onions, cooked	24	29	1.2	0.8	27	33	4 oz.
parsley, raw	204	63	0.3	3.2	58	18	1 oz.
pickles, dill or sour	26	21	0.8	1.2	29	24	4 oz.
potato, white	29	188	6.5	0.2	65	426	8 oz.
potato salad	19	63	3.3	0.3	22	72	4 oz.
romaine or leaf lettuce	68	25	0.4	2.7	77	28	4 oz.
sauerkraut, canned	36	18	0.5	2.0	41	20	4 oz.
spinach, steamed	93	38	0.4	2.4	105	43	4 oz.
squash, cooked	25	25	1.0	1.0	28	28	4 oz.
squash, uncooked	28	29	1.0	1.0	64	66	8 oz.
string beans	119	104	0.9	1.1	270	235	8 oz.
succotash, frozen	13	85	6.5	0.2	15	96	4 oz.
sweet potato, baked	40	58	1.5	0.7	91	132	8 oz.
sweet potato, candied	37	43	1.2	0.9	84	97	8 oz.
Swiss chard, steamed	73	24	0.3	3.1	83	27	4 oz.
tomato paste, canned	27	70	2.6	0.4	31	79	4 oz.
tomato puree, canned	13	34	2.7	0.4	29	77	8 oz.
tomato, canned	6	19	3.2	0.3	14	43	8 oz.
tomato, uncooked	13	27	2.1	0.5	15	31	4 oz.
vegetables, mixed frozen	29	74	2.5	0.4	33	83	4 oz.
yellow snap beans	56	43	0.8	1.3	64	49	4 oz.

GRAINS AND GRAIN PRODUCTS	mg per 100 grams		P/Ca	Ca/P	mg per serving		serving
	calcium	phosph.	(bad)	(good)	calcium	phosph.	size
bran flakes	53	358	6.8	0.1	60	405	4 oz.
brown rice, cooked	12	73	6.1	0.2	14	83	4 oz.
corn flakes	16	32	2.0	0.5	18	36	4 oz.
farina, instant	77	60	0.8	1.3	174	136	8 oz.
French bread	45	85	1.9	0.5	13	24	1 oz.
graham crackers	40	143	3.6	0.3	11	41	1 oz.
hamburger/hot dog buns	73	87	1.2	0.8	42	49	2 oz.
macaroni & cheese	181	161	0.9	1.1	410	365	8 oz.
oat meal, cooked	9	58	6.6	0.2	20	133	8 oz.
pancakes	220	338	1.5	0.7	499	766	8 oz.
pizza	221	195	0.9	1.1	502	442	8 oz.
pretzels	22	132	6.1	0.2	25	149	4 oz.
shredded wheat	43	389	9.1	0.1	49	441	4 oz.
spaghetti with meat sauce	50	95	1.9	0.5	113	216	8 oz.
toasted wheat germ	48	1085	22.7	0.0	54	1230	4 oz.
waffles	113	173	1.5	0.7	257	393	8 oz.
wheat bran	119	1121	9.4	0.1	135	1271	4 oz.
white bread, enriched	100	115	1.2	0.9	113	130	4 oz.
white rice, cooked	10	28	2.8	0.4	11	32	4 oz.
whole wheat flour	41	372	9.1	0.1	12	105	1 oz.

FRUITS	mg per 100 grams		P/Ca	Ca/P	mg per serving		serving
	calcium	phosph.	(bad)	(good)	calcium	phosph.	size
apples	7	10	1.4	0.7	16	23	8 oz.
apricots, dried	67	108	1.6	0.6	76	122	4 oz.
apricots, uncooked	17	34	2.0	0.5	19	38	4 oz.
avocado	10	42	4.1	0.2	23	96	8 oz.
banana	8	26	3.3	0.3	18	59	8 oz.
blueberries	15	13	0.9	1.2	17	15	4 oz.
cantaloupe	14	16	1.1	0.9	32	36	8 oz.
cherries	22	19	0.9	1.2	25	22	4 oz.
cranberries	124	20	0.2	6.2	140	23	4 oz.
dates, dried	59	63	1.1	0.9	67	71	4 oz.
figs, dried	124	76	0.6	1.6	140	86	4 oz.
grapefruit	18	18	1.0	1.0	40	40	8 oz.
grapes, green, seedless	8	13	1.6	0.6	18	29	8 oz.
lemons	17	11	0.6	1.6	20	12	4 oz.
olives, canned	106	17	0.2	6.2	120	19	4 oz.
orange	41	20	0.5	2.1	93	45	8 oz.
papaya	35	104	3.0	0.3	80	235	8 oz.
peach	9	19	2.2	0.5	20	44	8 oz.
pears, canned	5	7	1.4	0.7	6	8	4 oz.
pears, uncooked	8	11	1.3	0.8	19	25	8 oz.
pineapple	17	8	0.5	2.2	39	18	8 oz.
strawberries	21	21	1.0	1.0	24	24	4 oz.
tangerines	30	13	0.4	2.2	67	30	8 oz.
watermelon	7	10	1.4	0.7	16	23	8 oz.

MEATS	mg per 100 grams		P/Ca	Ca/P	mg per serving		serving
	calcium	phosph.	(bad)	(good)	calcium	phosph.	size
bacon, broiled or fried	14	224	16.1	0.1	16	254	4 oz.
bacon, Canadian	19	218	11.5	0.1	22	247	4 oz.
beef, pot roast or chuck roast	11	140	12.7	0.1	25	317	8 oz.
bologna	7	128	18.2	0.1	16	291	8 oz.
chicken chow mein	23	117	5.1	0.2	52	265	8 oz.
chicken liver, cooked	11	159	14.4	0.1	25	360	8 oz.
chicken, broiled	9	201	22.2	0.0	21	457	8 oz.
chicken, roast	11	265	24.0	0.0	25	602	8 oz.
chicken, fried	13	272	20.5	0.0	30	616	8 oz.
corned beef	9	93	10.3	0.1	21	211	8 oz.
frankfurter	5	102	20.1	0.0	12	231	8 oz.
hamburger	22	141	6.3	0.2	51	320	8 oz.
ham, cured, roast	9	172	19.5	0.1	20	390	8 oz.
lamb chops, broiled	9	156	17.7	0.1	20	354	8 oz.
pork chops, roast	10	232	23.4	0.0	23	526	8 oz.
steak, T-bone, porterhouse, rib	10	186	18.7	0.1	23	422	8 oz.
turkey, roast	11	300	27.2	0.0	25	680	8 oz.
TV dinner, meat loaf	19	117	6.1	0.2	43	265	8 oz.
TV dinner, turkey	37	124	3.4	0.3	84	281	8 oz.
veal cutlet, broiled	11	225	20.4	0.0	25	510	8 oz.

FISH AND SEAFOOD	mg per 100 grams		P/Ca	Ca/P	mg per serving		serving
	calcium	phosph.	(bad)	(good)	calcium	phosph.	size
crabmeat, canned	43	174	4.1	0.2	97	395	8 oz.
flounder, baked	23	349	14.9	0.1	53	792	8 oz.
halibut, broiled	16	252	15.4	0.1	37	571	8 oz.
kelp	1093	240	0.2	4.6	310	68	1 oz.
salmon, sockeye, canned	258	342	1.3	0.8	585	776	8 oz.
sardines, canned in oil	272	432	1.6	0.6	618	980	8 oz.
shrimp, cooked	72	190	2.6	0.4	163	431	8 oz.
tuna, canned in oil, drained	8	233	29.3	0.0	18	528	8 oz.

EGGS AND DAIRY PRODUCTS	mg per 100 grams		P/Ca	Ca/P	mg per serving		serving
	calcium	phosph.	(bad)	(good)	calcium	phosph.	size
cheese, American or cheddar	753	476	0.6	1.6	1708	1081	8 oz.
cheese, creamed cottage	94	152	1.6	0.6	214	345	8 oz.
cheese, parmesan	1143	782	0.7	1.5	1296	887	4 oz.
egg, raw, boiled, or poached	54	206	3.8	0.3	31	117	2 oz.
milk, human	33	13	0.4	2.5	76	30	8 oz.
skim milk	121	95	0.8	1.3	275	216	8 oz.
whole milk	118	93	0.8	1.3	267	210	8 oz.
yogurt, low-fat	120	94	0.8	1.3	272	213	8 oz.

SOUP	mg per 100 grams		P/Ca	Ca/P	mg per serving		serving
	calcium	phosph.	(bad)	(good)	calcium	phosph.	size
chicken noodle soup	4	15	3.8	0.3	9	34	8 oz.
ministrone	15	24	1.6	0.6	34	54	8 oz.
split pea soup	12	61	5.1	0.2	27	139	8 oz.

SAUCES AND CONDIMENTS	mg per 100 grams		P/Ca	Ca/P	mg per serving		serving
	calcium	phosph.	(bad)	(good)	calcium	phosph.	size
blackstrap molasses	685	85	0.1	8.1	194	24	1 oz.
French salad dressing	11	14	1.3	0.8	3	4	1 oz.
Italian salad dressing	10	4	0.4	2.5	3	1	1 oz.
kelp	1093	240	0.2	4.6	310	68	1 oz.
light molasses	165	45	0.3	3.7	47	13	1 oz.
maple syrup	105	8	0.1	13.1	30	2	1 oz.
mustard	124	134	1.1	0.9	35	38	1 oz.
soy sauce	82	104	1.3	0.8	23	29	1 oz.
tomato catsup	22	50	2.3	0.4	6	14	1 oz.

JUICES	mg per 100 grams		P/Ca	Ca/P	mg per serving		serving
	calcium	phosph.	(bad)	(good)	calcium	phosph.	size
apple juice	6	9	1.5	0.7	14	21	8 oz.
grapefruit juice	8	14	1.8	0.6	18	32	8 oz.
lemon juice	7	13	2.0	0.5	2	4	1 oz.
orange juice, fresh	11	17	1.5	0.7	25	39	8 oz.
orange juice, frozen concentrate	32	54	1.7	0.6	73	122	8 oz.
tomato juice	7	18	2.6	0.4	16	41	8 oz.

NUTS, SEEDS, AND NUT BUTTER	mg per 100 grams		P/Ca	Ca/P	mg per serving		serving
	calcium	phosph.	(bad)	(good)	calcium	phosph.	size
almonds, roasted and salted	234	504	2.2	0.5	266	572	4 oz.
cashews, unsalted	39	373	9.6	0.1	44	423	4 oz.
peanut butter	57	380	6.6	0.2	65	431	4 oz.
peanuts, roasted, salted	75	401	5.4	0.2	85	455	4 oz.
sesame seeds, whole	1160	616	0.5	1.9	1315	699	4 oz.
sesame seeds, hulled	110	592	5.4	0.2	125	671	4 oz.
sunflower seeds	120	837	7.0	0.1	136	949	4 oz.
walnuts	0	570		0.0	0	646	4 oz.

FRUITS	silicon mg per 100 grams
acerolas	7
apples	64
apricots	53
avocado	11
bananas	20
blackberries	51
blueberries	0
boysenberries	0
canteloupe	88
casaba	0
honeydew	0
muskmelon	88
cheries	66
coconut	88
cranberries	2
currants, black	20
dates	2
figs	35
lemons	4
limes	4
olives	7
oranges	4
papaya	4
peaches	2
pears	7
persimmons	0
plums	18
prunes	13
pomegranate	2
pumpkin	17
rasberries, black	18
rhubarb	2
strawberries	22
tangeriens	1
tomatoes	11
watermelon	11

VEGETABLES	silicon mg per 100 grams
alfalfa	0
artichokes	2
asperagus	2
beans, kidney	2
beans, lima	4
beans, string	2
beets	88
broccoli	22
brussels sprouts	2
cabbage	9
cabbage, savoy	104
carrots	22
cauliflower	33
celery	31
chard	7
corn	18
cucumbers	35
dandelion greens	135
eggplant	4
garlic	22
horseradish	225
kale	2
leeks	97
lettuce	86
lettuce, romaine	40
onions	99
parsley	38
parsnips	168
peas	2
bell peppers	33
potatoes, white	22
potatoes, sweet	20
radish	9
spinach	181
turnips	11

boron		
parts per million		
	lowest of several tests	highest of several tests
snap beans	10	73
cabbage	7	42
lettuce	6	37
tomatoes	5	36
spinach	12	88

REFERENCES
Chapter 1

1 Richards B; *Blood of the Moon*. ODAE Productions, Toronto, Ontario, 1992.

2 Utian, WH; Case Western Reserve Medical School, Cleveland.

3 Choay P; Lafond JL; Favier A. [Value of micronutrient supplements in the prevention or correction of disorders of menopause]. *Revue Francaise de Gynecologie et D Obstetrique*, 1990 Dec, 85(12):702-5.

4 Metka M. [Osteoporosis and estrogens]. *Wiener Med Wochenschrift*, 1990 Oct 15, 140(18-19):485-6.

5 Arnaud CD; Sanchez SD. The role of calcium in osteoporosis. *Annual Review of Nutrition*, 1990, 10:397.

6 Doren M; Schneider HP. Identification and treatment of postmenopausal women at risk for development of osteoporosis. *Intl of Clinical Pharmacology, Therapy, and Toxicology*, 1992 Nov, 30(11):431-3.

7 Lee, JR. *Optimal Health Guidelines*, 1991.

8 Editorial, *Lancet*, 1993, 341:151-2.

9 Ibid.

10 Ibid.

Chapter 2

1 Ho KK; Weissberger AJ. Impact of short-term estrogen administration on growth hormone secretion and action: distinct route-dependent effects on connective and bone tissue metabolism. *Journal of Bone and Mineral Research*, 1992 Jul, 7(7):821-7.

2 Balfour JA; Heel RC. Transdermal estradiol. A review of its pharmacodynamic and pharmacokinetic properties, and therapeutic efficacy in the treatment of menopausal complaints. *Drugs*, 1990, 40:561-82.

3 Di Carlo F. [Action of drugs in relation to the administration route]. *Mineral Endocrinology*, 1989 Jan-Mar, 14(1):41-4.

4 Balfour, op cit.

5 Di Carlo, op cit.

6 Goretzlehner G. [Efficacy of different estrogens as subject to mode of application (published erratum appears in Zentralbl Gynakol 1990;112:1248)]. Zentralblatt fur Gynakologie, 1989, 111:1093-100.

7 Ibid.

8 Vorster HH et al. Egg intake does not change plasma lipoprotein and coagulation profiles. *American Journal of Clinical Nutrition*, 1992 Feb, 55(2):400-10.

Chapter 3

1 *The Incredible Machine*, National Geographic Society, 1986, p 239.

2 Baird DT; Glasier AF. Drug Therapy: Hormonal Contraception. *NEJM*, 1993, 328:1543.

3 Kamen, B; *Everything You Always Wanted to Know About Potassium But Were Too Tired to Ask* (Novato, California: Nutrition Encounter, 1992).

4 Vasuvattakul Set al. Kaliuretic response to aldosterone: influence of the content of potassium in the diet. *American Journal of Kidney Diseases*, 1993 Feb, 21(2):152-60.

5 Rhofes, R; Pflanzer, R. *Human Physiology* (Fort Worth, Texas: Saunders College Publishing, Harcourt Brace, 1992), p 435.

6 Ibid, p 1015.

7 Richard Kunin, M.D. Personal communication, February 1, 1993.

8 Edgren RA. Clincial use of sex steroids, Year Book Medical Publishers, Inc., 1980.

9 Ibid.

10 Ibid.

11 Lee, op cit.

12 Ibid.

Chapter 4

1 Posting on the WELL, electronic communication, 1993. <Athena>.

2 Richards B; *Blood of the Moon*. ODAE Productions, Toronto, Ontario, 1992.

3 Seligmann J; Gelman D. Is it sadness or madness? *Newsweek*, March 15, 1993, p 66.

4 Rhofes, R; Pflanzer, R. *Human Physiology* (Fort Worth, Texas: Saunders College Publishing, Harcourt Brace, 1992), p 992.

5 Kamen B. *Everything You Always Wanted to Know About Potassium But Were Too Tired to Ask* (Novato, California: Nutrition Encounter, 1992).

6 Rosseel M; Schoors, D. Chewing gum and hypokalemia. *Lancet*, 1993, 341:175.

7 Lane JD; Steege JF; Rupp SL; Kuhn CM. Menstrual cycle effects on caffeine elimination in the human female. *European Journal of Clinical Pharmacology*, 1992, 43(5):543-6.

8 Shephard, BD; Shephard, CA. *Complete Guide to Women's Health* (NY: Penguin books, 1990), p 443.

9 Lever J; Brush MG. *Premenstrual Tension* (New York: McGraw Hill, 1981), p 146.

10 Seaman, B; Seamn G. *Women and the Crisis in Sex Hormones* (NY: Rawson Associates, 1977), p 142.

11 Stewart F et al. *My Body, My Health* (New York: John Wiley & Sons, 1979), p 387.

12 Lurie S; Borenstein R. The premenstrual syndrome. *Obstetric and Gynecology Survey*, 1990 Apr, 45(4):220-8.

13 Hsia LS; Long MH. Premenstrual syndrome. Current concepts in diagnosis and management. *Journal of Nurse-Midwifery*, 1990 Nov-Dec, 35(6):351-7.

14 Derzko CM. Role of danazol in relieving the premenstrual syndrome. *Journal of Reproductive Medicine*, 1990 Jan, 35(1 Suppl):97-102.

15 Mansfield MJ; Emans SJ. Anorexia nervosa, athletics, and amenorrhea. *Pediatric Clinics of North America*, 1989 Jun, 36(3):533-49.

16 Ibid.

17 Fong AKH; Kretsch MJ. Changes in dietary intake, urinary nitrogen, and urinary volume across the menstrual cycle. *American Journal of Clinical Nutrition*, 1993, 57:43-6.

18 Rossignol AM; Bonnlander H. Prevalence and severity of the premenstrual syndrome. Effects of foods and beverages that are sweet or high in sugar content. *Journal of Reproductive Medicine*, 1991 Feb, 3:131-6.

19 Rabin DS et al. Hypothalamic-pituitary-adrenal function in patients with the premenstrual syndrome. *Journal of Clinical Endocrinology and Metabolism*, 1990 Nov, 71(5):1158-62.

20 Schweiger U et al. Caloric intake, stress, and menstrual function in athletes. *Fertility and Sterility*, 1988 Mar, 49(3):447-50.

21 Hesla JS et al. Superoxide dismutase activity, lipid peroxide production and corpus luteum steroidogenesis during natural luteolysis and regression induced by oestradiol deprivation of the ovary in pseudopregnant rabbits. *Journal of Reproduction and Fertility*, 1992 Aug, 95(3):915-24.

22 Caufriez A. Menstrual disorders in adolescence: pathophysiology and treatment. *Hormone Research*, 1991, 36(3-4):156-9.

23 Ibid.

Chapter 5

1 Burckhardt P; Michel C. The peak bone mass concept. *Clinical Rheumatology*, 1989 Jun, 8 Suppl 2:16.

2 Metzger DA; Hammond CB. Are estrogens indicated for the treatment of postmenopausal women? *Drug Intelligence and Clinical Pharmacy*, 1988 Jun, 22(6):493-6.

3 Ellis JM et al. A deficiency of vitamin B6 is a plausible molecular basis of the retinopathy of patients with diabetes mellitus. *Biophysical Research Communications*, 1991 Aug 30, 179(1):615-9.

4 Bernstein AL. Vitamin B6 in clinical neurology. *Annals of the New York Academy of Science*, 1990, 585:250-60.

5 Pascual E et al. Higher incidence of carpal tunnel syndrome in oophorectomized women. *British Journal of Rheumatology*, 1991 Feb, 30(1):60-2.

6 Zamboni M et al. Body fat distribution in pre- and post-menopausal women: metabolic and anthropometric variables and their inter-relationships. *International Journal of Obesity*, 1992 Jul, 16(7):495-504.

7 Matthews KA et al. Influences of natural menopause on psychological characteristics and symptoms of middle-aged healthy women. *Journal of Consulting and Clinical Psychology*, 1990 Jun, 58(3):345-51.

8 van Beresteyn EC; van t Hof MA; De Waard H. Contributions of ovarian failure and aging to blood pressure in normotensive perimenopausal women: a mixed longitudinal study. *American Journal of Epidemiology*, 1989 May, 129(5):947-55.

9 Hafner H et al. Oestradiol enhances the vulnerability threshold for schizophrenia in women by an early effect on dopaminergic neurotransmission. Evidence from an epidemiological study and from animal experiments. *European Archives of Psychiatry and Clinical Neuroscience*, 1991, 241(1):65-8.

10 Metzger DA; Hammond CB. Are estrogens indicated for the treatment of postmenopausal women? *Drug Intelligence and Clinical Pharmacy*, 1988 Jun, 22(6):493-6.

11 Fugere P. [Replacement hormone therapy: the earlier the menopause, the greater the importance of treatment (interview)]. *Union Medicale du Canada*, 1992 Mar-Apr, 121(2):125-9.

12 Kin K et al. Bone mineral density of the spine in normal Japanese subjects using dual-energy X-ray absorptiometry: effect of obesity and menopausal status. *Calcified Tissue Int*, 1991 Aug, 49:101.

13 Beard MK. Atrophic vaginitis. Can it be prevented as well as treated? *Postgraduate Medicine*, 1992 May 1, 91:257.

14 Zaridze D et al. Diet, alcohol consumption and reproductive factors in a case-control study of breast cancer in Moscow. *International Journal of Cancer*, 1991 Jun 19, 48(4):493-501.

15 Cummings SR et al. Bone density at various sites for prediction of hip fractures. *Lancet*, 1993, 341:72-5.

16 Prior JC; Vigna YM; Alojado N. Progesterone and the prevention of osteoporosis. *Canadian Journal of Obstetrics and Gynecology & Women's Health Care*, 1991, 3:178-84.

17 Leidy LE. Early age at menopause among left-handed women. *Obstetrics and Gynecology*, 1990 Dec, 76(6):1111-4.

18 Tajtakova M et al. [The effect of smoking on menopause *Journal of Obesity*, 1992 Jul, 16(7):495-504.

28 Roberts PJ, op cit.

Chapter 6

1 Kelly PJ; Eisman JA; Sambrook PN. Interaction of genetic and environmental influences on peak bone density. *Osteoporosis International*, 1990 Oct, 1(1):56-60

2 Hirota T et al. Effect of diet and lifestyle on bone mass in Asian young women. *American Journal of Clinical Nutrition*, 1992 Jun, 55(6):1168-73.

3 Tylavsky FA et al. Familial resemblance of radial bone mass between premenopausal mothers and their college-age daughters. *Calcified Tissue International*, 1989 Nov, 45(5):265-72.

4 Pollitzer WS; Anderson JJ. Ethnic and genetic differences in bone mass: a review with a hereditary vs environmental perspective [published erratum appears in American Journal of Clinical Nutrition, 1990 Jul;52(1):181]. *American Journal of Clinical Nutrition*, 1989 Dec, 50(6):1244-59.

5 Rhofes, R; Pflanzer, R *Human Physiology* (Fort Worth, Texas: Saunders College Publishing, Harcourt Brace, 1992), p 915.

6 Burton, BT. *Human Nutrition* (New York: McGraw-Hill, 1976), p 129.

7 Nordin BEC et al. Calcium and bone metabolism in old age. *Nutrition in Old Age*, ed Carlson LA (Uppsala, Sweden: Swedish Nutrition Foundation, 1972).

8 Albanese AA. *Current Topics in Nutrition and Disease*, vol 3 *Nutrition for the Elderly* (NY: Alan R Liss, Lutwak L. Continuing need for dietary calcium through life. *Geriatrics*, 1974, 29:171.

9 Macy IG. *Nutrition & Chemical Growth in Childhood* (Springfield, IL: Charles C Thomas, 1942).

10 Lees B et al. Differences in proximal femur bone density over two centuries. *Lancet*, 1993, 341:673:675.

11 Cummings SR et al. Bone density at various sites for prediction of hip fractures. *Lancet*, 1993, 341:72-5.

12 Caffeine causes loss of calcium from bone. *Calcified Tissue International*, 1992 Dec, 51(6):424-8.

13 Burckhardt P; Michel C. The peak bone mass concept. *Clinical Rheumatology*, 1989 Jun, 8 Suppl 2:16-21.

14 Kelly PJ; Eisman JA; Sambrook PN. Interaction of genetic and environmental influences on peak bone density. *Osteoporosis International*, 1990 Oct, 1(1):56-60.

15 Kritz-Silverstein D; Barrett-Connor E; Hollenbach KA. Pregnancy and lactation as determinants of bone mineral density in postmenopausal women. *American Journal of Epidemiology*, 1992 Nov 1, 136(9):1052.

16 Lutwak, op cit.

17 Ibid.

18 Ibid

19 Kamen B. *Startling New Facts About Osteoporosis* (Novato, California: Nutrition Encounter, 1992).

20 Nilsson BE; Westlin NE. Changes in bone mass in alcoholics. *Clinical Orthopedics and Related Research*, 1973, 90:229-32.

21 Meghji S. Bone remodelling. *British Dental Journal*, 1992 Mar 21, 172(6):235-42.

22 Ericson JE; Smith DR; Flegal AR. Skeletal concentrations of lead, cadmium, zinc, and silver in ancient North American Pecos Indians. *Environmental Health Perspectives*, 1991 Jun, 93:217-23.

23 Saltzman BE et al. Total body burdens and tissue concentrations of lead, cadmium, copper, zinc, and ash in 55 human cadavers. *Environmental Research*, 1990 Aug, 52(2):126-45.

24 Lee JR. *Optimal Health Guidelines*, 1991.

Chapter 7

1 Lee, J.R. Hormonal and Nutritional Aspects of Osteoporosis, *Health and Nutrition*, Vol 6, 1991, p 4.

2 Slootweg MC et al. Oestrogen and progestogen synergistically stimulate human and rat osteoblast proliferation. *Journal of Endocrinology*, 1992 May, 133(2):R5-8.

3 Tremollieres F; Pouilles JM; Ribot C. [Postmenopausal bone loss. Role of progesterone and androgens]. *Presse Medicale*, 1992 Jun 6, 21(21):989-93.

4 Hedlund LR; Gallagher JC. The effect of age and menopause on bone mineral density of the proximal femur. *Journal of Bone and Mineral Research*, 1989 Aug, 4(4):639-42.

5 Amano K et al. [Effect of suppletory estrogen or 1,25(OH)D3 on bone mineral content]. Nippon Sanka Fujinka Gakkai Zasshi. *Acta Obstetrica et Gynaecologica Japonica*, 1992 Jul, 44(7):833-6.

6 Hedlund LR; Gallagher JC., op cit.

7 National Institute of Health, Consnesus Conference: Osteoporosis, *Journal of the American Medical Association* 252 (1984):799.

8 Lee, J.R. Hormonal and Nutritional Aspects of Osteoporosis, *Health and Nutrition*, Volume 6, 1991, p 4.

9 Booher DL. Estrogen supplements in menopause. *Cleveland Clincal Journal of Medicine*, 1990 Mar-Apr, 57(2):15.

10 Cummings SR et al. Bone density at various sites for prediction of hip fractures. *Lancet*, 1993, 341:72-5.

11 Love RR et al. Effects of tamoxifen on bone mineral density in postmenopausal women with breast cancer. *New England Journal of Medicine*, 1992, 326:852-6.

12 Wisneski LA. Clinical management of postmenopausal osteoporosis. *Southern Medical Journal*, 1992 Aug, 85:832-9.

13 Clark AP; Schuttinga JA. Targeted estrogen/progesterone replacement therapy for osteoporosis: calcula tion of health care cost savings. *Osteoporosis International*, 1992 Jul, 2(4):195-200.

14 *Osteoporosis International* (8)

15 John Lee, personal communication, March, 1993.

16 Metka M. [Osteoporosis and estrogens]. *Wiener Medizinische Wochenschrift*, 1990 Oct 15, 140:485-6.

17 Lutwak L. Continuing need for dietary calcium through life. *Geriatrics*, 1974, 29:171.

Chapter 8

1 Electronic mail on The Well with Professor William H Calvin, University of Washington, January, 1993.

2 Forbes AP. Fuller Albright. His concept of postmenopausal osteoporosis and what came of it. *Clinical Orthopaedics and Related Research*, 1991 Aug(269):128-41.

3 "National Institute of Health, Consnesus Conference: Osteoporosis," *Journal of the American Medical Association* 252 (1984):799.

4 Lee, L. Estrogen, Progesterone and Female Problems. *Earthletter*, Vol. 1 no. 2, June 1991, p 1.

5 Reinisch JM; Sanders SA. Effects of prenatal exposure to diethylstilbestrol (DES) on hemispheric laterality and spatial ability in human males. *Hormones and Behavior*, 1992 Mar, 26(1):62-75.

6 Reinisch JM; Ziemba-Davis M; Sanders SA. Hormonal contributions to sexually dimorphic behavioral development in humans. *Psychoneuroendocrinology*, 1991, 16(1-3):213-78.

7 Telang NT et al. Induction by estrogen metabolite 16 alpha-hydroxyestrone of genotoxic damage & aberrant proliferation in mouse mammary epithelial cells. *Journal of the National Cancer Institute.*, 1992 Apr, 84:634.

8 Schlehofer B; Blettner M; Wahrendorf J. Association between brain tumors and menopausal status. *Journal of the National Cancer Institute*, 1992 Sep 2, 84(17):1346-9.

9 Burgat V. [Residues of drugs of veterinary use in food]. *Revue du Praticien*, 1991 Apr 11, 41(11):985-90.

10 Witkamp RF; Korstanje C; van Miert AS. [Toxicological and pharmacological effects of the use of bovine somatotropin in dairy farming]. *Tijdschrift voor Diergeneeskunde*, 1990 Sep 1, 115(17):780-8.

11 Nagasawa H. Physiological significance of hormones and related substances in milk with special reference to prolactin: an overview. *Endocrine Regulations*, 1991 Jun, 25(1-2):90-7.

12 Karg H. [The current status and risk evaluation of the use of hormone preparations in food producing animals]. *Monatsschrift Kinderheilkunde*, 1990 Jan, 138(1):2-5.

13 Moishezon-Blank N. Commentary on the possible effect of hormones in food on human growth. *Medical Hypotheses*, 1992 Aug, 38(4):273-7.

14 Ibid.

15 Gambrell RD Jr. Use of progestogens in postmenopausal women. *International Journal of Fertility*, 1989 Sep-Oct, 34(5):315-21.

16 Markovitz JH et al. Psychological, biological and health behavior predictors of blood pressure changes in middle-aged women. *Journal of Hypertension*, 1991 May, 9(5):399-406.

17 Kamen, B. *Startling New Facts About Osteoporosis* (Novato, CA: Nutrition Encounter).

18 Hermier D et al. Alterations in plasma lipoproteins and apolipoproteins associated with estrogen-induced hyperlipidemia in the laying hen. *European Journal of Biochemistry*, 1989 Sep 1, 184(1):109-18.

19 Wells, RG. "Should All Postmenopausal Women Receive Hormone Replacement Therapy?" *Senior Patient* 1 (1989):65

20 Kamen, B. *New Facts About Fiber* (Novato, California: Nutrition Encounter, 1991), p 47, quoted from the *Scandinavian Journal of Clinical and Laboratory Investigation,* 1990.

21 Whitehead MI; Hillard TC; Crook D. The role and use of progestogens. *Obstetrics and Gynecology,* 1990 Apr, 75(4 Suppl):59S-76S.

22 Henderson BE; Bernstein L. The international variation in breast cancer rates: an epidemiological assessment. *Breast Cancer Research and Treatment,* 1991 May, 18 Suppl 1:S11-7.

23 Ibid.

24 Key TJ; Pike MC. The role of oestrogens and progestagens in the epidemiology and prevention of breast cancer. European *Journal of Cancer and Clinical Oncology,* 1988 Jan, 24(1):29-43.

25 White JO et al. The human squamous cervical carcinoma cell line, HOG-1, is responsive to steroid hormones. *International Journal of Cancer,* 1992 Sep 9, 52(2):247-51.

26 Adams JB. Enzymatic regulation of estradiol-17 beta concentrations in human breast cancer cells. *Breast Cancer Research and Treatment,* 1992 Mar, 20(3):145-54.

27 Cantor KP; Lynch CF; Johnson D. Bladder cancer, parity, and age at first birth. *Cancer Causes and Control,* 1992 Jan, 3(1):57-62.

28 Chen A; Huminer D. The role of estrogen receptors in the development of gallstones and gallbladder cancer. *Medical Hypotheses,* 1991 Nov, 36(3):259-60.

29 Cagle PT; Mody DR; Schwartz MR. Estrogen and progesterone receptors in bronchogenic carcinoma. & colorectal cancer cell lines. *Cancer,* 1989 Jun 1, 63(11):2148-51.

32 Colin C. [Hormone substitution therapy in menopause and risk of breast cancer]. *Revue Francaise de Gynecologie et D Obstetrique, 1991* Jan, 86(1):27-8.

33 Reinisch JM; Sanders SA. Effects of prenatal exposure to diethylstilbestrol (DES) on hemispheric laterality and spatial ability in human males. Hormones and Behavior, 1992 Mar, (1):62-75.

Chapter 9

1 Lee, J.R. Hormonal and Nutritional Aspects of Osteoporosis, *Health and Nutrition,* Volume 6 issue 4, winter 1991, p 4.

2 Prior, J.C; Vigna, Y.; Alojada, N. Progesterone and the Prevention of Osteoporosis. *Canadian Journal of Ob/Gyn & Women's Health Care,* Volume 3, Number 4, 1991, p 181.

3 Prior, JC; Wark, JD; Barr, SI. The prevention and treatment of osteoporosis. *Lancet,* 1993, 328:65-6.

4 Tremollieres F; Pouilles JM; Ribot C. [Postmenopausal bone loss. Role of progesterone and androgens]. *Presse Medicale,* 1992 Jun 6, 21(21):989-93.

5 Lee, J. Is Natural Progesterone the Missing Link in Osteoporosis Prevention and Treatment? *Medical Hypotheses* (1991) 35, 316-318.

6 Coen D; Terzian E; Magrini N. The prevention and treatment of osteoporosis. *Lancet,* 1993, 328:65-6.

7 Gallagher JC; Golder D; Kabie WT. 1986. Effects of Therapy Vary on Different Parts of the Skelaton. *Clinical Research* 34:927A.

8 Gallagher JC; Golder D; Kabie WT. 1986. Comparison of Estrogen and Progestin therapy on cortical and trabecular bone using spa, dpa and qct. *XX Int Nat Conf CT.*

9 Prior, J.C. Progesterone as a Bone-Trophic Hormone *Endocrine Reviews,* Vol. 11 No. 2, 1990 p 394.

10 Peat, R. *Nutrition for Women,* Lake Oswego, Oregon (Centotech, 1981) p 25-26.

11 Hargrove, J et al. Menopausal Hormone Replacement Therapy With Continuous Daily Oral Micronized Estradiol and Progesterone. *Obstetrics & Gynecology,* Vol 73 No 4, April 1989.

12 Personal interview with Martin Milner, N.D., January 14, 1993, Las Vegas.

13 Ibid.

14 Prior JC. Progesterone as a bone-trophic hormone. Endocrine Reviews, 1990 May, 11(2):386-98.

15 Barengolts EI et al. Effects of progesterone on postovariectomy bone loss in aged rats. *Journal of Bone and Mineral Research,* 1990 Nov, 5(11):1143-7.

16 Lindsay R. The effect of sex steroids on the skeleton in premenopausal women. *American Journal of Obstetrics and Gynecology,* 1992 Jun, 166(6 Pt 2):1993-6.

17 Prior JC. Progesterone as a bone-trophic hormone. *Endocrine Reviews,* 1990 May, 11(2):386-98.

18 Ibid.

19 Lindsay R. The effect of sex steroids on the skeleton in premenopausal women. *American Journal of Obstetrics and Gynecology,* 1992 Jun, 166(6 Pt 2):1993-6.

20 Blaakaer J et al. The pituitary-gonadal axis in women with benign or malignant ovarian tumors. *Acta Endocrinologica,* 1992 Aug, 127(2):127-30.

Chapter 10

1 Eaton SB; Nelson DA. Calcium in evolutionary perspective. *American Journal of Clinical Nutrition* 1991,54:Suppl:281S-7S.

2 Heany, R.P. "Thinking straight about calcium." *New England Journal of Medicine*, 1993, 328:503-5.

3 Lees B et al. Differences in proximal femur bone density over two centuries. *Lancet*, 1993, 341:673:675.

4 Op cit, Heany.

5 Ettinger B. Role of calcium in preserving the skeletal health of aging women. *Southern Medical Journal*, 1992 Aug, 85(8):2S22-30.

6 Angus RM et al. Dietary intake and bone mineral density. *Bone and Mineral*, 1988 Jul, 4(3):265-77.

7 De Lucas, H. The Lastt Information on Vitamin D and Bone Status. *Complimentary Medicine* (1986):13.

8 Heikinheimo RJ et al. Annual injections of vitamin D and fractures of aged bones. *Calcification Tissue International*, 1992, 327:1637-42.

9 *British Medical Journal* 289 (1984):1103.

10 Chalmers, J. Geographical Variations in Senile Osteoporosis. *Journal of Bone and Joint Surgery* 52B (1970):667.

11 Charles P. Calcium absorption and calcium bioavailability. *Journal of Internal Medicine*, 1992 Feb, 231(2):161-8.

12 Strain JJ. A reassessment of diet and osteoporosis—possible role for copper. *Medical Hypothesis*, 1988 Dec, 27(4):333-8.

13 Reid IR et al. Effect of calcium supplementation on bone loss in postmenopausal women. *New England Journal of Medicine*, 1993, 328:460-4.

14 Cummings SR et al. Bone density at various sites for prediction of hip fractures. *Lancet*, 1993, 341:72-5.

15 Metka M. [Osteoporosis and estrogens]. *Wiener Medizinische Wochenschrift*, 1990 Oct 15, 140(18-19):485-6.

16 Arnaud CD; Sanchez SD. The role of calcium in osteoporosis. *Ann Rev of Nutrition*, 1990, 10:397-414.

17 Fujita T; Fukase M. Comparison of osteoporosis and calcium intake between Japan and the United States. *Proceedings of the Society for Experimental Biology and Medicine*, 1992 Jun, 200(2):149-52.

18 Riis, B; Thomsen, K; Christiannsen, C. Does Calcium Supplementation Prevent Postmenopausal Bone Loss? *New England Journal of Medicine* 316(1987):173.

19 Sheikh, MS et al, "Gastrointestinal Absorption of Calcium from Milk and Calcium Salts," *New England Journal of Medicine* 317 (1987):532.

20 Stevenson, JC. "Dietary Calcium and Hip Fracture," *Lancet* 2(1988):1318.

21 Dudl, RJ et al, Evaluation of Intravenous Calcium Therapy for Osteoporosis, *American Journal of Medicine* 55(1973):631.

22 Strier KB. Menu for a monkey. *Natural History*, 1993, 102:34-42.

Chapter 11

1 Recker, RR, "The Effect of Milk Supplements on Calcium Metabolism, Bone Metabolism, and Calcium Balance," *American Journal of Clinical Nutrition* 41 (1968):254.

2 Sheehy, G. *The Silent Passage*, (New York, Random House, 1992) p 103.

3 *Journal of Clinical Pediatric Dentistry*, 1991, 16:38.

4 *Roczniki Panstwowego Zakladu Higieny*, 1989, 40:266.

5 Lee, J.R. Hormonal and Nutritional Aspects of Osteoporosis. *Health and Nutrition*, 1991, 6:7.

6 Riggs BL et al. Effect of Flouride Treatment on Fracture Rate in Postmenopausal Women with Osteoporosis. *New England Journal of Medicine*, 1990, 322:802-9.

7 Sowers, FR et al. A Prospective Study of Bone Mineral Content and Fracture in Communities with Differential Flouride Exposure. *American Journal of Epidemiology*, 1991, 133:649-660.

8 Jacobsen, SJ et al. Regional Variation in the Incidence of Hip Fracture. *Journal of the American Medical Association*, 1990, 264:500-502.

9 Cooper C et al. Water Flouridation and Hip Fracture. *Journal of the American Medical Association*, 1991, 266:513.

10 Danielson C. *Journal of the American Medical Association*, August 12, 1992.

11 Randal J. USA: Another flap over fluoride. *Lancet*, 1990, 335:282.

12 Revis. Chlorinated drinking water and reduced calcium intake enhance the hypercholesterolemic effect of high fat diet. *Clinical Research*, 1983, 31:865.

13 Report issued by North Marin Water District, Novato, California, 1991.

14 Arnaud CD; Sanchez SD. The role of calcium in osteoporosis. *Ann Rev of Nutr*, 1990, 10:397-414.

15 Rader JI. Anti-nutritive effects of dietary tin. *Advances in Exp Medicine and Biology*, 1991, 289:509-24.

16 Alfrey A. Aluminum intoxication. *New England Journal of Medicine,* 1983.

17 Kiiskinen A; Heikkinen E. Effect of prolonged physical training on the development of connective tissues. In *Metabolic Adaptation to Prolonged Physical Exercise.* Eds Howald H and Poortmans JR (Basel: Birkhauser Verlag, 1975), pp 253-61.

18 Steinhaus AH. Chronic effects of exercise. *Physiological Reviews*, 1933, 13:103-47.

19 Heavy caffeine use linked to increased hip fractures. *Am Jnl of Epid*, 1990 Oct, 132(4):675-84.

20 Caffeine causes loss of calcium from bone.*Calcified Tissue International*, 1992 Dec, 51(6):424-8.

21 Hunt IF; Murphy NJ; Henderson C. Food and nutrient intake of Seventh-day Adventist women. *American Journal of Clinical Nutrition*, 1988 Sep, 48(3 Suppl):850-1.

22 Hunt IF; Murphy NJ; Henderson C. Food and nutrient intake of Seventh-day Adventist women. *American Journal of Clinical Nutrition*, 1988 Sep, 48(3 Suppl):850-1.

23 Marsh AG et al. Vegetarian lifestyle and bone mineral density. *American Journal of Clinical Nutrition*, 1988, 48:837.

24 Pouilles JM; Tremollieres F; Ribot C. [Comparative effects of sodium fluoride and hormonal replacement therapy on bone metabolism in osteoporotic women with high fracture risk. Results of monitoring for 2 years]. *Revue du Rhumatisme et des Maladies Osteo-Articulaires*, 1992 Feb, 59(2):103-13.

25 Haddock DA. A simple way to manage menopause. *Postgraduate Medicine*, 1990 Sep 1, 88(3):131-5, 138.

26 Burckhardt P; Michel C. The peak bone mass concept. *Clinical Rheumatology*, 1989, 8 Suppl 2:16-21.

27 Kelly PJ; Eisman JA; Sambrook PN. Interaction of genetic and environmental influences on peak bone density. *Osteoporosis International*, 1990 Oct, 1(1):56-60.

28 Seelig MS. The requirement of magnesium by the normal adult. *AJCN,* 1964, 14:342-90.

29 Prior JC; Vigna YM; McKay DW. Reproduction for the athletic woman. New understandings of physiology and management. *Sports Medicine*, 1992 Sep, 14(3):190-9.

30 Strain JJ. A reassessment of diet and osteoporosis—possible role for copper. *Medical Hypotheses*, 1988 Dec, 27(4):333-8.

31 Prince RL et al. Prevention of postmenopausal osteoporosis. A comparative study of exercise, calcium supplementation, and hormone-replacement therapy. *New England Journal of Medicine*, 1991 Oct 24, 325(17):1189-95.

Chapter 12

1 Personal interviews with Robert Cathcart, M.D., 1990-93, San Francisco.

2 Nordin BE; Morris HA. Osteoporosis and vitamin D. *Journal of Cellular Biochemistry*, 1992 May, 49(1):19-25.

3 Lee, J.R. Hormonal and Nutritional Aspects of Osteoporosis. *Health and Nutrition*, 1991, 6:7.

4 Johnson K; Kligman EW. Preventive nutrition: disease-specific dietary interventions for older adults. *Geriatrics*, 1992 Nov, 47(11):39-40, 45-9.

5 Lee. Op cit.

6 Kamen B. *Osteoporosis: What It Is, How to Prevent It, How to Stop It* (New York: Pinnacle, 1984), p 102.

7 Kunin RA. *Mega-Nutrition for Women* (New York: McGraw-Hill, 1983), p 159.

8 Gogu SR et al. Protection of zidovudine-induced toxicity against murine erythroid progenitor cells by vitamin E. *Experimental Hematology*, 1991 Aug, 19(7):649-52.

9 Kaufmann K. *Silica: The Forgotten Nutrient* (British Colombia, Canada: Alive Books, 1990).

10 Pennington JA. Silicon in foods and diets. *Food Additives and Contaminants*, 1991 Jan-Feb, 8(1):97-118.

11 Villareal CP; Juliano BO. Variability in contents of thiamine and riboflavin in brown rice, crude oil in brown rice and bran-polish, and silicon in hull of IR rices. *Plant Foods for Human Nutrition*, 1989 Sep, 39:287.

12 Nielsen, FH et al. Boron enhances and mimics some effects of estrogen therapy in postmenopausal women. *Journal of Trace Elements and Experimental Medicine*, 1992, 5:237-46.

13 Hunt CD; Shuler TR; Mullen LM. Concentration of boron and other elements in human foods and personal-care products. *Journal of the American Dietetic Association*, 1991 May, 91(5):558-68.

14 Mann J; Inman W. Oral contraceptives and death from myocardial infarction. *British Medical Journal,* 1975, 2:841. 15 Kamen B. *The Chromium Diet, Supplement & Exercise Strategy* (Novato, CA: Nutrition Encounter, 1990).

16 Raisz LG; Kream BE. Regulation of bone formation. Part 2. *New England Journal of Medicine*, 1983, 309:83-9.

17 *Cancer Letters*, 1992 Oct 21, 66(3):207-16.

18 *Carcinogenesis*, 1992 Oct, 13(10):1847-51.

19 Babal K. *Nutrition and Meganutrients* (Los Angeles, 1993).

20 Personal interview, Martin Milner, N.D., Las Vegas, 1993.

21 Choay P; Lafond JL; Favier A. [Value of micronutrient supplements in the prevention or correction of disorders accompanying menopause]. *Rev Francaise de Gyn et D Obstetrique*, 1990 Dec, 85(12):702-5.

22 Benova DK. Anticlastogenic effects of a polyvitamin product, 'Pharmavit', on gamma-ray induction of somatic and germ cell chromosome aberrations in the mouse. *Mut Res*, 1992 Oct, 269(2):251-8.

23 Franceschi RT. The role of ascorbic acid in mesenchymal differentiation. *Nutrition Reviews*, 1992 Mar, 50(3):65.

24 Khan PK; Sinha SP. Antimutagenic efficacy of higher doses of vitamin C. *Mut Res*, 1993 Jan, 298:157.

25 Lupulescu A. Ultrastructure and cell surface studies of cancer cells following vitamin C administration. *Experimental and Toxicologic Pathology*, 1992 Mar, 44(1):3-9.

26 Ghosh A; Sharma A; Talukder G. Relative protection given by extract of Phyllanthus emblica fruit and an equivalent amount of vitamin C against a known clastogen—caesium chloride. *Food and Chemical Toxicology*, 1992 Oct, 30(10):865-9.

27 Franceschi RT. The role of ascorbic acid in mesenchymal differentiation. *Nutrition Reviews*, 1992 Mar, 50(3):65.

28 Eisele PH et al. Skeletal lesions and anemia associated with ascorbic acid deficiency in juvenile rhesus macaques. *Laboratory Animal Care*, 1992 Jun, 42(3):245-9.

29 Arnaud CD; Sanchez SD. The role of calcium in osteoporosis. Ann Rev of Nutr, 1990, 10:397-414.

30 Cruz ML et al. Effect of chronic maternal dietary magnesium deficiency on placental calcium transport. *Journal of the American College of Nutrition*, 1992 Feb, 11(1):87-92.

31 Rubinacci A et al. [Influence of nutrition, age and vitamin D status on fasting urinary excretion of calcium in postmenopausal women]. *Minerva Medica*, 1992 Oct, 83(10):601-8.

32 Khaw KT; Sneyd MJ; Compston J. Bone density parathyroid hormone and 25-hydroxyvitamin D concentrations in middle aged women. *British Medical Journal*, 1992 Aug 1, 305(6848):273-7.

33 Charles P. Calcium absorption and calcium bioavailability. *Journal of Internal Medicine*, 1992 Feb, 231(2):161-8.

34 Hamilton SJ; Buhl KJ. Acute toxicity of boron, molybdenum, and selenium to fry of chinook salmon and coho salmon. *Archives of Environmental Contamination and Toxicology*, 1990, 19:366-73.

35 Nielsen FH et al. Magnesium and methionine deprivation affectthe response of rats to boron deprivation. *Biological Trace Element Research*, 1988, 17:91-107.

36 Nielsen, FH. New essential trace elements for the life sciences. *Bio Trace El Res*, 1990, 26-27:599-611.

37 Nielsen FH. Ultratrace minerals mythical elixirs or nutrients of concern? Boletin - *Asociacion Medica de Puerto Rico*, 1991 Mar, 83(3):131-3.

38 Newnham RE. Agricultural practices affect arthritis. *Nutrition and Health*, 1991, 7(2):89-100.

39 Leicht E; Biro G. Mechanisms of hypocalcaemia in the clinical form of severe magnesium deficit in the human. *Magnesium Research*, 1992 Mar, 5(1):37-44.

40 Seelig MS. The requirement of magnesium by the normal adult. *American Journal of Clinical Nutrition*, 1964, 14:342-90.

41 Mancinella A.[Silicon, a trace element essential for living organisms. Recent knowledge on its preventive role in atherosclerotic process, aging and neoplasms]. *Clinica Terapeutica*, 1991 Jun 15, 137(5):343-50.

42 Carlisle EM. Silicon as a trace nutrient. *Science of the Total Environment*, 1988 Jul 1, 73(1-2):95-106.

Chapter 13

1 Khashaeva TKh; Magataeva MN; Tsadkina GG. [Clinico-immuno-hormonal parallels in obese women in the climacteric period]. *Akusherstvo i Ginekologiia*, 1991 Jul(7):59-63.

2 Schoutens A et al. Serum triiodothyronine, bone turnover, and bone mass changes in euthyroid pre- and postmenopausal women. *Calcified Tissue International*, 1991 Aug, 49(2):95-100.

3 Koga M; Nakao H; Sato B. Effects of retinoic acid on estrogen- and thyroid hormone-induced growth in a newly established rat pituitary tumor cell line. *Journal of Steroid biochemistry & Molecular Biochemistry*, 1992 Oct, 43:263.

4 Maruo T et al. A role for thyroid hormone in the induction of ovulation and corpus luteum function. *Hormone Research*, 1992, 37 Suppl 1:12-8.

5 Forsyth IA. The mammary gland. *Baillieres Clinical Endocrinology and Metabolism*, 1991 Dec, 5,:809.

6 Matsuo H et al. [Modification of endocrine function of trophoblasts by thyroid hormone]. Nippon Sanka Fujinka Gakkai Zasshi. *Acta Obstetrica et Gynaecologica Japonica*, 1991 Nov, 43(11):1533-8.

7 Martinez, M; Derksen D; Kapsner P. Making sense of hypothyroidism. *Postgrad Med*, 1993, 93(6):135.

8 Urban RJ. Neuroendocrinology of aging in the male and female. *Endocrinology and Metabolism Clinics of North America*, 1992 Dec, 21(4):921-31.

9 Martinez, M; Derksen D; Kapsner P. Making sense of hypothyroidism. *Postgraduate Medicine*, 1993, 93(6):135.

10 Rosen CJ; Adler RA. Longitudinal changes in lumbar bone density among thyrotoxic patients after attainment of euthyroidism. *Jnl of Clinical Endocrinology and Metabolism*, 1992 Dec, 75(6):1531-4.

11 Coindre JM et al. Bone loss in hypothyroidism with hormone replacement: a histomorphometric study. *Archives of Internal Medicine*, 1986, 146(1):48-53.

12 Stall GM et al. Accelerated bone loss in hypothyroid patients overtreated with L-thyroxine. *Annals of Internal Medicine*, 1990, 113(4):265-9.

13 Franklyn JA et al. Long-term thyroxine treatment and bone mineral density. *Lancet*, 1992 Jul 4, 340:9-13.

14 Kronfol Z. Stress and immunity. *Lancet*, 1993, 341:881-2.

15 Kovalenko AN; Sushko VA; Fedirko MI. [The hormonal functions regulating carbohydrate metabolism in participants in the cleanup of the sequelae of the accident at the Chernobyl Atomic Electric Power Station with a neurocirculatory dystonia syndrome]. *Vrachebnoe Delo*, 1992 Jun(6):52-5.

16 Kamen B. *Osteoporosis: What It Is, How to Prevent It, How to Stop It* (New York: Pinnacle, 1984). p 36.

17 Moyers, op cit.

18 Verma S et al. Superoxide dismutase activation in thyroid and suppression in adrenal. Novel pituitary regulatory routes. *Febs Letters*, 1991 May 6, 282(2):310-2.

19 McMahon A et al. Regulation of tyrosine hydroxylase and dopamine beta-hydroxylase mRNA levels in rat adrenals by a single and repeated immobilization stress. *Journal of Neurochemistry*, 1992 Jun, 58(6):2124-30.

20 Salieva RM et al. Delta sleep-inducing peptide as a factor increasing the content of substance P in the hypothalamus and the resistance of rats to emotional stress. *Neurosci & Beh Res*, 1992 Jul-Aug, 22:275.

21 Kiseleva ZM. [Effect of emotional stress on catecholamine and dopa levels in some central nervous regions and in the heart of experimental animals]. *Kardiologiia*, 1992 May, 32(5):81-4.

22 deCatanzaro D; Macniven E. Psychogenic pregnancy disruptions in mammals. *Neuroscience and Biobehavioral Reviews*, 1992 Spring, 16(1):43-53.

Chapter 14

1 Dalton, KD, *Once a Month* (Pomona CA, Hunter House, 1979) p 178.

2 Wiklund I et al. Long-term effect of transdermal hormonal therapy on aspects of quality of life in postmenopausal women. *Maturitas*, 1992 Mar, 14(3):225-36.

3 Robert Atkins, M.D. Personal interview, January 29, 1993.

4 Lauersen NH. *Natural Progesterone* (New York).

5 Lee JR. Osteoporosis reversal with trnasdermal progesterone. *Lancet*, 1990, 336:1327.

6 Lee JR. Is natural progesterone the missing link in osteoporosis prevention and treatment? *Medical Hypothesis*, 1991, 35:316-18.

7 Dalton, op cit.

8 Colditz GA et al. Type of postmenopausal hormone use and risk of breast cancer: 12-year follow-up from the Nurses' Health Study. *Cancer Causes and Control*, 1992 Sep, 3(5):433-9.

9 Personal communication - Dr. Lee.

10 Letter from Esther M. Kirk, M.D., Westwood Village, November 1984.

11 Letter from Louis J. Marx. M.D., March 1984.

12 Richard Kunin, M.D. Personal communication, February 1, 1993.

13 Letter from John R. Lee, M.D., April 1984.

14 Storch M; Carmichael C. *How to Relieve Cramps and other Menstrual Problems* (NY: Workman Publishing, 1982), p 49.

15 Dalton K. Prenatal Progesterone and Educational Attainments. *British Journal of Psychiatry*, 1976, 129:438-42.

16 Reinisch JM; Ziemba-Davis M; Sanders SA. Hormonal contributions to sexually dimorphic behavioral development in humans. *Psychoneuroendocrinology,* 1991, 16(1-3):213-78.

17 Foresta C et al. Progesterone induces capacitation in human spermatozoa. *Andrologia*, 1992 Jan-Feb, 24(1):33-5.

18 Ben-Nun I et al. Therapeutic maturation of endometrium in in vitro fertilization and embryo transfer. *Fertility and Sterility*, 1992 May, 57(5):953-62.

19 National Geographic, October 1992. Lee, John, M.D. Personal interview, February 11, 1993.

20 Giamarchi D et al. [Bronchial hyperreactivity in non-asthmatic patients harboring a uterine fibroma]. *Allergie et Immunologie*, 1989 Feb, 21(2):72-5.

21 Dalton, KD, *Once a Month* (Pomona CA, Hunter House, 1979) p 53.

22 Herzog AG. Reproductive endocrine considerations and hormonal therapy for women with epilepsy. *Epilepsia*, 1991, 32 Suppl 6:S27-33

23 Tauboll E; Lindstrom S. The effect of progesterone and its metabolite 5 alpha-pregnan-3 alpha-ol-20-one on focal epileptic seizures in the cat's visual cortex in vivo. *Epilepsy Research*, 1993 Jan, 14(1):17-30.

24 Lee, John, M.D. Personal communication. Letter, December 11, 1992.

25 Hargrove JT et al. Menopausal hormone replacement therapy with continuous daily oral micronized estradiol and progesterone. *Obstetrics & Gynecology*, 1989, 73:606-12.

26 Wu ZY; Wu XK; Zhang YW. Relationship of menopausal status and sex hormones to serum lipids and blood pressure. *International Journal of Epidemiology*, 1990 Jun, 19(2):297-302.

27 Crane Mg; Harris JJ; Winsor W II. Hypertension, oral contraceptive agents, and conjugated estrogesn. *Annals of Internal Medicine*, 1971:74:13-21.

28 Robert Atkins, M.D. Personal interview, January 29, 1993.

29 Riis BJ et al. The effect of percutaneous estradiol and natural progesterone on postmenopausal bone loss. *American Journal of Obstetrics and Gynecology*, 1987, 156:61-5.

30 Shaaban MM. Contraception with progestogens and progesterone during lactation. *Journal of Steroid Biochemistry and Molecular Biology*, 1991, 40(4-6):705-10.

31 Norman RJ et al. Inhibin and relaxin concentrations in early singleton, multiple, and failing pregnancy: relationship to gonadotropin and steroid profiles. Jan, 59(1):130-7.

32 Segal S; Casper RF. Progesterone supplementation increases luteal phase endometrial thickness and oestradiol levels in in-vitro fertilization. *Human Reproduction*, 1992 Oct, 7(9):1210-3.

33 Laurikka-Routti M; Haukkamaa M; Lahteenmaki P. Suppression of ovarian function with the transder mally given synthetic progestin ST 1435. *Fertility and Sterility*, 1992 Oct, 58(4):680-4.

34 Baird DT. Clinical use of mifepristone (RU 486). *Annals of Medicine*, 1993 Feb, 25(1):65-9.

35 Elks ML. Peripheral effects of sex steroids: implications for patient management. *Journal of the American Medical Womens Association*, 1993 Mar-Apr, 48(2):41-6, 50.

36 Sitruk-Ware R. Percutaneous and transdermal oestrogen replacement therapy. *Annals of Medicine*, 1993 Feb, 25(1):77-82.

37 Ibid.

38 Ibid.

39 Sitruk-Ware R. Estrogen therapy during menopause. Practical treatment recommendations. *Drugs*, 1990 Feb, 39(2):203-17.

40 Jordan VC et al. The estrogenic activity of synthetic progestins used in oral contraceptives. *Cancer*, 1993 Feb 15, 71(4 Suppl):1501-5.

Chapter 15

1 Baker DP. Estrogen-replacement therapy in patients with previous endometrial carcinoma. *Comprehensive Therapy*, 1990 Jan, 16(1):28-35.

2 Willett WC et al. Intake of *trans* fatty acids and risk of coronary heart disease among women. *Lancet*, 1993, 341:581-5.

3 Froom J. Selections from current literature: hormone therapy in postmenopausal women. *Family Practice*, 1991 Sep, 8(3):288-92.

4 Schlemmer A et al. Urinary magnesium in early postmenopausal women. Influence of hormone therapy on calcium. *Magnesium and Trace Elements*, 1991-92, 10(1):34-9.

5 Henderson BE; Bernstein L. The international variation in breast cancer rates: an epidemiological assessment. *Breast Cancer Research and Treatment*, 1991 May, 18 Suppl 1:S11-7.

6 Cummings SR. Evaluating the benefits and risks of postmenopausal hormone therapy. *American Journal of Medicine*, 1991 Nov 25, 91(5B):14S-18S.

7 Steingold KA et al. Comparison of transdermal to oral estradiol administration on hormonal and hepatic parameters in women with premature ovarian failure. *Journal of Clinical Endocrinology and Metabolism*, 1991 Aug, 73(2):275-80.

8 Balfour JA; Heel RC. Transdermal estradiol. A review of its pharmacodynamic and pharmacokinetic properties, and therapeutic efficacy in the treatment of menopausal complaints. *Drugs*, 1990 Oct, 40:561.

9 Wiklund I et al. Long-term effect of transdermal hormonal therapy on aspects of quality of life in postmenopausal women. *Maturitas*, 1992 Mar, 14(3):225-36.

10 Kirkham C et al. A randomized, double-blind, placebo-controlled, cross-over trial to assess the side effects of medroxyprogesterone acetate in hormone replacement therapy. *Obstetrics and Gynecology*, 1991 Jul, 78(1):93-7.

11 Testimony presented to FDAs Fertility and Maternal Health Drugs Advisory Committee, June, 1992.

12 Ibid.

13 Cundy T. *British Medical Journal*, July 6, 1991.

14 Stehlin D. Depo-provera: the quarterly contraceptive. *FDA Consumer*, 1993, 27:11-13.

15 Metzger DA; Hammond CB. Are estrogens indicated for the treatment of postmenopausal women? *Drugs*.

16 Backstrom T; Hammarback S. Premenstrual syndrome—psychiatric or gynaecological disorder? *Annals of Medicine*, 1991 Dec, 23(6):625-33.

17 Ibid.

18 Leather AT; Savvas M; Studd JW. Endometrial histology and bleeding patterns after 8 years of continuous combined estrogen and progestogen therapy in postmenopausal women. *Obstetrics and Gynecology*, 1991 Dec, 78(6):1008-10.

19 Wiklund I; Holst J; Karlberg J; Mattsson LA; Samsioe G; Sandin K; Uvebrant M; von Schoultz B. A new methodological approach to the evaluation of quality of life in postmenopausal women. *Maturitas*, 1992 Mar, 14(3):211-24.

20 Amano K; Nemoto R; Kato Y; Masuda R; Nishijima M. [Effect of suppletory estrogen or 1,25(OH)D3 on bone mineral content]. Nippon Sanka Fujinka Gakkai Zasshi. *Acta Obstetrica et Gynaecologica Japonica*, 1992 Jul, 44(7):833-6.

21 Wolf PH et al. Reduction of cardiovascular disease-related mortality among postmenopausal women who use hormones: evidence from a national cohort. *American Journal of Obstetrics and Gynecology*, 1991 Feb, 164(2):489-94.

22 Konner M. *Medicine at the Crossroads* (New York: Pantheon Books, 1993), p 75.

23 Schneider HP; Doren M. [Osteoporosis from the gynecologic viewpoint]. *Zentralblatt fur Gynakologie*, 1992, 114(7):333-50.

24 Baum E. [Psychosocial effects of the onset of menopause and physical symptoms in early postmenopause]. *Psychotherapie, Psychosomatik, Medizinische Psychologie*, 1990 Jun, 40(6):200-6.

25 Ferguson KJ; Hoegh C; Johnson S. Estrogen replacement therapy. A survey of women's knowledge and attitudes. *Archives of Internal Medicine*, 1989 Jan, 149(1):133-6.

26 Schlemmer A et al. Urinary magnesium in early postmenopausal women. Influence of hormone therapy on calcium. *Magnesium and Trace Elements*, 1991-92, 10(1):34-9.

27 Reinisch JM; Ziemba-Davis M; Sanders SA. Hormonal contributions to sexually dimorphic behavioral development in humans. *Psychoneuroendocrinology*, 1991, 16(1-3):213-78.

28 Doren M; Schneider HP. Identification and treatment of postmenopausal women at risk for the development of osteoporosis. *International Journal of Clinical Pharmacology, Therapy, and Toxicology*, 1992 Nov, 30(11):431-3.

29 Lindsay R. The effect of sex steroids on the skeleton in premenopausal women. *American Journal of Obstetrics and Gynecology*, 1992 Jun, 166(6 Pt 2):1993-6.

30 Lindsay R. The effect of sex steroids on the skeleton in premenopausal women. *American Journal of Obstetrics and Gynecology*, 1992 Jun, 166(6 Pt 2):1993-6.

31 Sitruk-Ware R. Percutaneous and transdermal oestrogen replacement therapy. *Annals of Medicine*, 1993 Feb, 25(1):77-82.

32 Jordan VC et al. The estrogenic activity of synthetic progestins used in oral contraceptives. *Cancer*, 1993 Feb 15, 71(4 Suppl):1501-5.

33 Felson DT et al. The effect of postmenopausal estrogen therapy on bone density in elderly women. *New England Journal of Medicine*, 1993, 329:1141-6.

34 Ibid.

35 Nordon BE et al. The relative contribution of age and years since menopause to postmenopausal bone loss. *Journal of Clinical Endocrinology Metabolism*, 1990, 70:83-88.

36 Heany RP. Estrogen-calcium interactions in the postmenopause: a quantitative description. *Bone Mineral*, 1990, 11:67-84.

37 Eisenberg DM et al. Unconventional medicine in the United States: prevavlennce, costs, and patterns of use. *New England Journal of Medicine*, 1993, 328:246-52.

I N D E X